Simple Steps to a Longer Life

The 6 Pillars of Staying Healthy Forever

Dr. Jason Plotsky

Dedication

For you, Dad. Thank you for the life lessons
and providing me with my why.

Acknowledgments

This book wouldn't have happened without seeing devoted patients over my last twenty-plus years of chiropractic practice. Your questions drove me to research concepts and try to provide the best possible answers to your health issues. Those of you who had to work hard to get rid of years of pain and dysfunction proved to me that these concepts work in real life. You have shown me not to give up hope and to trust in the power of the human body.

Most importantly, I would like to thank my wife, Cindy, for taking such great care of our boys and teaching them the concepts from the book. You walk the walk, day in and day out. Thank you for sharing my vision of increasing the health consciousness of our community. Also, thank you for being patient with me over the last three years while I worked on this book.

To my three boys: David, Alex, and Peyton. You are true blessings in my life. You helped me create a bigger *why* for myself. I hope this book provides a framework for you to stay healthy for the rest of your lives. May you find your passion in life as I have mine. Discover your unique gifts and talents, and find a way to be of service to others.

I would like to thank my mom for her never-ending love and support. Thank you, Mom, for all of the vitamins and cooking lessons and for acting as my personal taxi. I can still remember going to the health food store and buying the peanut butter you had to stir! I look forward to having the same mental sharpness as you at the age of eighty!

Thank you to my sister, Jodi. I have nothing but positive memories from our time growing up together. You were always there for me, especially when we lost our father. You are an excellent mother, and I cherish the time we have spent together.

And, of course, this book is dedicated to my late father, David Plotsky. While he left us way too early, he provided guiding principles I will never forget: Do things that matter. Leave a lasting impression. Follow your dreams. And most importantly, take care of your body; it's the only one you get.

To my team at Nova Spinal Care, past and present: Thank you for providing excellent service to our patients and helping me teach some of the principles in this book. I can't do my job without your support, and I have been fortunate to always have great people around me. Also, thank you to those of you working in the background, behind the camera, helping me with my social media and making memorable events.

To my in-laws, Linda and Conrad Toner, thank you for raising amazing human beings! The two of you have been great role models for those in their seventies and eighties. You've always shown that aging is a mindset, and you have proven that consistency is the key to health.

To the medical professionals, researchers, and health influencers who work hard to create content, write books, and promote healthy living, I know what a tireless and never-ending job this can be, but your contributions do make a difference. Keep it up!

I would like to acknowledge the work of my first editor, Miriam. Thank you for getting me started on this journey and helping me get the rough manuscript together.

To my editor, Cierra Lamb, thank you for believing in this project and helping me articulate my thoughts in a clear and concise manner. This wouldn't have been possible without your attention to detail and your editorial expertise.

Finally, thank you to the team at Superior Book Productions for getting this book completed (finally) and into a place for the world to see.

Contents

Introduction

"You've got to call your mother right now—something's happened to your dad."

I was working in the clinic and in my last semester of chiropractic school at the time, and my girlfriend—who eventually became my wife—had relayed the message to me. I lived about three blocks away from school, so I frantically ran home and called my mom.

"Your dad is very sick..." she began.

I didn't really understand what that meant, even when the doctors repeated it in a subsequent conversation. Dad was never sick—he was an optometrist and had never missed a day of work. Never in his whole life. I never saw him sick. He was never hurt. He could always work. He even coached baseball in his spare time. I just couldn't imagine what "very sick" meant since those words and my dad did not belong in the same sentence.

"...he had a heart attack."

ii Dr. Jason Plotsky ~ Simple Steps to a Longer Life

Okay, I thought. "Lots of people have heart attacks," I said.

"No, Jason. He's...he's really sick. You need to come here, like, right now."

I was in Iowa then, and my parents were on vacation in Florida. Just three short weeks before, we had been together for Christmas. In fact, we'd recently discussed whether my dad would ever slow down. He was sixty-two, and I thought he should take it easy and enjoy life a bit more.

"Why would I slow down now?" he had replied. "I'm at the peak of my career. New patients are referred to me all the time. I am super-busy, and I love what I do...."

I replayed this conversation over and over again in my mind, interspersed with my mother's voice saying, "Your dad is very sick...." I flew to Florida and drove a rental car through the night straight to the hospital.

As I entered the room, I surveyed all the machines responsible for monitoring, feeding, and keeping my father alive; he was unconscious and unaware of any of them. My knees buckled, I hit the floor, and I just lost it. My mother and sister were there and patiently let me have that moment.

"Is...is...is he going to wake up? He's going to be okay, right?" I didn't know if I was asking a question or issuing a command. And no one knew the answer to that at the time. It was a waiting game.

In the morning, the cardiologist repeated the same line: "Your dad is really sick." It was as though the universe were intent on that sinking in with me, and I still couldn't grasp it.

Trying to visualize my father being sick was impossible. Even now, after I had actually seen him in such a state, it was difficult to wrap my mind around it.

The cardiologist continued. "There is a good chance if your dad makes it through this, he won't be able to walk down to get the mail."

A pulmonologist joined us, repeated what the cardiologist said, and then added, "If he doesn't come around soon, he will not survive without the machines."

It was far worse than I'd thought. We had a difficult decision to make.

They unplugged the machines, and I watched my dad take his last breath. I never had an opportunity to speak with him one more time, never got to hug him one last time, nor had a chance to get his advice.

After that short moment, that was it.

The impact, however, was felt by many for many years.

Longevity Isn't Ethereal

Many of us like the idea of a long, quality life, but few of us understand our health's effect on others. We might look at our children and grandchildren and think, "I hope I'm around to see them _____," filling in the blank with various milestones like graduating from high school, launching a career, getting married, having children, and so on. We don't consider the effect it might have on them if we don't see them achieve those milestones. Or how difficult it will be for them to achieve those milestones if we hang around in poor health, requiring their care.

Instead, we relegate good health and longevity to the recesses of our minds, leaving it to "genetics" and luck instead of recognizing that, to a large extent, we have the power to control much of it. We might resolve each year on January 1 to turn our health around—we'll read a book, follow a friend's advice, maybe even go to the gym—and by Valentine's Day, we revert back to our genetics-and-luck plan, never fully addressing why we give up or why we wanted to improve our health in the first place.

Perhaps some of you are bristling, "Hey—I do prioritize my health," thinking a salad once a week for lunch proves your point...or maybe you really do understand what "prioritizing your health" means, but you aren't sure how to take it to the next level.

Others may feel overwhelmed by information or have experienced some symptoms and figure, "There's a pill I can take for that." Maybe you no longer have the amount of flexibility you once had, have gained weight you can't seem to lose, or certain foods affect you differently now—so you resign yourself, thinking, *It just comes with age.*

If any of these—or a combination of these—sounds like what's been stirring in your head, keep reading.

"But I Don't Feel Sick!"

The most obvious assumption people make is, "If I'm not sick, then I'm healthy." In our minds, we may justify that because we have no major health issues or aren't experiencing any pain or symptoms, we're good. We may even joke with friends, "Life's not worth living without [insert favorite food indulgence here]!"

A lack of symptoms is not the definition of health; one does not cancel out the other. My dad owned a business with dozens of employees, and my mother was a stay-at-home mom when we were young. Dad had felt fine the last time we spoke, and his death made an immediate and long-term impact on all of us, emotionally and financially. As much as I loved my father and he loved us, I doubt he thought much about whether he needed to take a deeper dive into his own health for the sake of us—if he felt fine, then he must be healthy, right? I can guarantee you that a week before he had his fatal heart attack, he felt good.

And my father isn't alone.

An estimated 70 percent of North Americans will be diagnosed with a chronic disease by age sixty-five. The most common chronic diseases are what I call "The Big Four"— cancer, diabetes, neurodegenerative diseases/dementia, and cardiovascular disease. Seventy percent is a big number, and I'd wager a large portion of that percentage experienced a "sudden" onset, having few to no symptoms before their diagnosis.

What's more likely is they had a chronic condition called metabolic syndrome, a cluster of three or more conditions (abdominal obesity, high blood pressure, high blood sugar, high triglyceride levels, low HDL, or "good" cholesterol) that increase a person's risk of developing one of the Big Four. It was like they "felt fine," so they didn't take those conditions as seriously as they should have.

But judging your overall health by how you feel now is a bad plan.

I don't state that to strike fear and paranoia into you, but that 70 percent statistic should alert you that most of us are in similar, ticking-time-bomb situations—even if we appear healthy on the outside and the numbers in our blood work fall within healthy ranges. We are heart attacks waiting to happen, we have cancer that is silently taking over our bodies, or we may soon have issues with our insulin levels.

We aren't able to see the disease that's brewing inside of us, so we keep doing the things we always do, making the same decisions we've always made and assuming they have no effect on our overall health because we don't *feel* sick.

I will say it again: Judging your overall health by how you feel now is a bad plan.

And it may be the biggest mistake you can make.

Good health isn't just luck or genetics. While you can't escape your physiology or biology, your body will always react to its environment. It can only handle so much stress, whether that stress is external or self-inflicted. We can take simple, concrete actions to correct what we are doing to ourselves, actions that don't require hours in the gym or eating only lettuce for the rest of our lives.

What Do We Trust?

A lot of claims are made about what makes us healthy. Haven't we all chuckled at the fact that soft drinks were initially promoted as health drinks? And we know which one was originally produced with cocaine, right? If you've been around for even the past twenty years, you've seen a lot of trends. The Information Age allows just about anyone with Wi-Fi to position themselves as a health guru. In these scenarios, the winning trends are the ones that have the most clicks, shares, and savviest press relations...not necessarily the most accurate information. In an attempt to stay relevant and cutting edge, accuracy is waived by way of a disclaimer's fine print.

As someone who understands science and physiology, I still struggle to filter down to what is true and to understand the source of and motivation behind information.

Finding true, unbiased sources of information is very difficult. And it's unfortunate when our healthcare providers and the pharmaceutical industry are blended in with this landscape of information because the perspective can be skewed. I'm not saying healthcare providers can't be true sources, but I am saying you need to consider the perspective and the lens through which they are viewing an issue.

I've had patients who don't understand they are victims of polypharmacy. Their pain began with, for example, lower back issues, so they were prescribed an anti-inflammatory drug. Then, they start having stomach issues, so they need a "stomach pill" to calm it down, many of them unaware that it's a known side effect of their anti-inflammatory prescription. And on it goes, but my main concern is that these sorts of drugs were never intended for long-term use.

And it's not just limited to prescribed medications. Many over-the-counter medications may be recommended for chronic issues without considering how it may affect other organs, like the kidneys or liver. Common, seemingly safe meds are recommended for long-term use and shouldn't be; patients are not really trained to ask questions like:

- Is it safe, long-term?
- What other effects will it have on my body?
- Are there any other organs or systems that this could be detrimental to?

We don't think to ask those questions because we just want to be rid of the pain. Our society trends toward seeing something in the media, asking your doctor, and taking it as truth. It's worse in the United States than it is in Canada, where I live, because those types of commercials are not aired as often here.

There is no way they have done studies on the effects of these multiple medications on people long-term. Who would sign up for that study? If someone came up to you and said, "We want you to take this anti-inflammatory drug, this stomach pill, this blood pressure pill, and this statin; we'll follow you for the next five years and see what happens with that combination of drugs," you would run in the opposite direction. When the drugs are added over time, however, we deduce that since each medication is safe to use on its own, it must be fine in combination. But we don't actually know that because those studies haven't been done.

We're taught to trust everything our providers tell us is true, and whether we want to admit it or not, we also trust what we see in the media we consume, whether it's televisions, magazines, or even social media. In doing so, we trust biased sources with an agenda.

Wait—I Have an Agenda, Too

We live in a symptom-suppression society, one that is trained to take any noticeable symptom and immediately try to suppress it instead of getting to the root of it. We immediately reach for relief for minor aches and ailments without stopping to think that maybe our body is intelligent enough to respond (with pain, fever, etc.) for a very good reason.

Part of my job as a practitioner is to ask questions like, "Why do you think you have headaches? Is it because you have an aspirin deficiency? Is that why your back hurts? Do you have a [insert name of anti-inflammatory drug] deficiency?"

When I ask these questions, most people will think for a second, and then respond, "No I don't have a deficiency." So why do you think you have pain, then? Why do you think you have inflammation? No one asks those questions to drill down to the root problem.

So, in full transparency…I have an agenda, too.

I want to make sure you understand the consequences of what you put into your body and what you expose it to. When we only treat symptoms, we ignore the signals our bodies send us.

My agenda also includes hope.

Inflammation is at the core of the Big Four and other chronic conditions like metabolic syndrome. By addressing the inflammation, I have seen heart disease and Type 2 diabetes literally reversed. I have witnessed others fight cancer successfully without chemotherapy and different types of drugs, and others work themselves out of a health crisis by doing the opposite of what they were doing to get there in the first place. These lifestyle diseases can be slowed, halted, or even reversed—without spending hours in the gym, in the kitchen, or giving up your favorite dessert.

Some scientists have estimated we know only 20 percent about how the body works, with the brain being the most complicated frontier. As a practitioner, I don't assume I know everything—I am constantly learning more and more about how the body works. The landscape changes as our world and society change.

Consider how the environmental impact on our bodies has changed dramatically in the last hundred years; back then, fewer cars were on the road, and there was more green space, better soil, and less pollution. There is a flipside to this; back then, fewer laws were in place to protect our food from contamination, littering was common, and smoking still wasn't connected to cancer. As we learn, however, we can modify our lifestyle to produce the response that we're looking for in the body.

My agenda for you, then, is to help you understand what is normal in your body and how it works. That way, when you have symptoms, you know that your body is trying to tell you something. Your first instinct will be to treat a symptom as an indicator that needs your attention rather than to mask it.

I also want to help you understand that you have a massive influence on how well your body works by changing the input. Your daily lifestyle choices not only affect how well your body works today but also in the future. You'll learn about some of the small changes I made, which made all the difference, but more importantly, we'll figure out what sorts of small changes you can make to reverse the bad, promote the good, and keep your health thriving.

This Is Not Another Health Book

I can't force you to make these changes, nor do I want to overwhelm you to the point you shut down. I'm not going to suggest you stop eating chips forever or start jogging three miles a day, every day. All that does is yield discouragement and disappointment. Even if you can keep that up for a week or two, it's not realistic to think you won't hit a stumbling block at some point.

The third part of my agenda involves making a plan for when you hit that stumbling block—because even if you stumble, that doesn't mean you have to fall. And if you fall, you don't have to stay down.

What's in This Book

This book has two parts. Part One focuses on your mindset and motivation—this is the key to making long-term changes and doing hard things. We'll walk through how to arrive at your *why* and its ability to leverage your success. Your ability to get through Part Two of this book will rest solely on the strength of your *why*, so don't skip ahead—work through Part One.

Part Two contains what I refer to as The Six Pillars of Health. Most of these are the likely suspects—food, sleep, movement, and so on—but the information is based on my own research and twenty years in clinical practice (personally and professionally). All of the pillars need your attention in order to benefit your overall health. The order in which you prioritize that attention will be suggested based on what I have found to have the greatest effect.

Good health isn't a given, and each of us has a different path to getting to our optimal state. But the sooner we turn on the switch and make better decisions regarding our health, the easier and more affordable it is to attain it.

This book will help you pinpoint what you'll need to do to accomplish your health goals, but I am certain it won't require hours in the gym or in the kitchen. Your strategy doesn't have to be perfect; it just needs to be leveraged to keep you moving forward.

It won't happen in a week. If you're looking for instant change, this isn't the book for you. You might be successful that first week and perhaps even the second, but I want you to make small, gradual changes that lead to long-term success. Leveraging your *why* will create small behavioral changes that lead to better and better outcomes. Turn the page, prepare to dig deep, and let's begin building toward lasting change.

PART I:

Getting to *Why*

Look, there are a lot of days I don't feel like exercising. If you followed me around for a week, you wouldn't be impressed by the hours a day I spend in the gym or kitchen (because I don't, in either setting). There are plenty of evenings after work that it would be far easier for me to pull through a drive-thru and pick up dinner than actually prepare a meal at home. If you run into me at the grocery store, you might see stuff in my cart that doesn't exactly fall into the "good for you" category. I'm not ashamed of it. I don't profess to do everything perfectly 100 percent of the time. I just know what that stopping point is for me.

My body needs to stick to my strategy 90 percent of the time to keep it in peak condition. So yes, I have my slacker moments, but having learned how to leverage my *why*, I have more successful days than not.

Your body is so intelligent it will do whatever it can to respond to your input, whether positive or negative. What we want, ultimately, are positive outcomes—good health now, good health later, and the type of longevity that's accompanied by a good quality of life (because what is the point of longevity if you spend that time hooked up to machines?).

But before you take that action, you must know your deepest reasons for wanting to take it in the first place. You need to get really clear on the outcome you want, and create leverage for why you *must* do it. That means eliminating wishful thinking and the shoulda-coulda-wouldas—i.e., I really should exercise and change my diet; if I did, I could run that 5k with my daughter, and I would feel like traveling more—and flip the switch that connects your mind to your actions.

I figured out the things I need to do regularly and consistently to keep my body working optimally. I know I can keep moving forward if I adhere to my strategy 90 percent of the time.

We'll figure out your stopping point in a later chapter, but right now, we need to identify what will motivate you to keep moving forward, particularly when you don't want to.

Striving for perfection will quickly wear you out. Don't worry. This discussion is not about making you choose between misery and failure—there is no quality in life if your options consistently leave you feeling deprived.

We have to be realistic with our goals. Speaking as someone whose children are active in travel sports, I know those days when your dinner becomes items off a fast-food menu because it's getting later and later, and everyone is hangry.

This process is not about perfection or restriction—it is about action. You can make many, many decisions throughout your day for the sake of your health...but your *why* will give you that extra nudge on those days when the choices are more difficult.

CHAPTER 1

The Problem

If you'd asked him, my father would have said he considered himself a healthy person, mainly because he felt fine and was rarely home sick. His heart attack was not because he had crazy cholesterol—it happened because he was an untreated type 2 diabetic, and his blood sugar remained consistently high and damaged the vessels in his heart. When they looked at his kidneys and some of the other organs and systems affected by his diabetes, other changes were already in progress, too, because of his high blood sugar. His diet was the primary culprit, but he also had other lifestyle flaws. I don't think he ever connected those dots between his weight, his diabetes, and his heart.

My father's death was part of a metabolic wake-up call for me. A few months after Dad passed away, I moved to Whidbey Island on the coast of Seattle for my internship. I was cooking for myself, but not exercising much, and overall, I just didn't feel great. I was avoiding fast food, but I still managed to put on about ten to fifteen pounds! I wasn't pounding the chocolate bars...but I was eating a lot of pasta and sandwiches, thinking I was eating healthy. That weight gain was the next part of the wake-up call. Something clicked, and I decided if I wanted to change my destiny, I had to formulate a short list of things to make it happen.

I started reading books and studies on metabolic health and followed some of the leading scientists in the field. While most of us have been programmed to think our health and longevity are largely determined by genetics, more and more evidence proves lifestyle choices have a larger influence. I was consumed with questions: What is the best diet for losing weight? What's the best way to reverse heart disease? How can I optimize my blood sugar? What is the secret among people who live the longest in the world? What common traits do they have?

Sure, genetics plays a role. When I speak to groups, I often tell them I probably have the worst genes in the room in terms of heart health, metabolic health, and longevity. When you make the connection between your habits and your desired long-term outcome, however, it creates some leverage for you to correct some of the weak spots your genetics have given you.

In this chapter, we'll look at some mindset, lifestyle, and situational factors that contribute (or don't) to your overall health.

Change Your Identity

In the introduction, I mentioned what I call The Big Four of chronic illnesses: Type 2 diabetes, heart disease, cancer, and neurodegenerative disease/dementia. I also mentioned metabolic syndrome, a chronic condition that often precedes the Big Four. All of these have major lifestyle factors involved, and they are mostly preventable (or at a minimum, we can delay their onset).

When I conduct workshops, I always ask the audience, "What would happen if you were not around?" Then I ask them to look at the person on their left and right and tell them, "At least one of you will be diagnosed with a lifestyle-related chronic disease by age sixty-five...likely, it will be cancer, heart disease, diabetes, or dementia."

The response is almost always the same: "But they're able to screen for these better now. They are detecting cancer sooner; screening for these things has come a long way and is far more sophisticated."

That's probably true to a certain extent. But if you just look at pictures of people from the 1960s-1970s, people, including athletes, were a lot thinner than they are now. So, beyond the more sophisticated screenings, I will ask them, "What else has changed in the past hundred years? Have our genes changed?" Then, the crowd falls silent until someone meekly says, "Honestly, I don't know the answer to that." No one really considers it.

(The answer is "No," by the way. Our genes have not changed.)

The answer is lifestyle.

Your body is designed to be healthy, but so many things can go wrong. And yes, some rare, genetic-related diseases can affect a very small percentage of us. I'm not addressing those individuals; I'm addressing the rest of us, the majority of us who have some control over The Big Four. Your body is designed to be healthy, but it can only handle so much of a poor diet, lack of movement, high stress, and lack of sleep before those things start to have an effect.

Most of us aren't thinking about the long-term effect of our short-term choices. At the time of writing, my father-in-law is in his late seventies. He still runs and does push-ups and chin-ups...for him, that is who he is. It is his mindset, his identity, where he says, "I am a runner, and I am a fit person." It is at his core; it's simply who he is.

Many of us marvel at seniors who are still fit. They're featured on the news or become subjects of documentaries. The rest of us are in awe, wondering how they are able to fit in exercise. Why, at their age, do they make that a priority? Because each of them has identified themselves as a fit and healthy person. As a result, the choices they make are those of a fit and healthy person.

Most people do not identify themselves as a person who will age well; instead, they accept that they are getting stiffer and slower and their bodies are wearing down with age. A lot of my patients are hoping to do things in the future without any concrete plan for how that will happen. We make assumptions that our mobility will be there when we need it, but every day, I am taking care of people who wish they could turn back the clock and start doing more for themselves sooner.

My whole practice is based on changing this mindset. No matter your starting point, if you start to implement the things we know can make a difference, you can decrease a lot of aging's effects. You can still increase your range of motion and mobility. Through lifestyle modifications—nothing extreme—you can reduce your inflammation, which is linked to so many chronic illnesses. I have many patients who, by making small changes, no longer need to take various medications, including prescriptions for arthritis and diabetes.

What changed in each of these cases was their *identity*. They found a reason to change and develop a mindset that they were going to be someone new, someone different than the person who resigned and submitted to aging.

The Silent Symptoms

The term "silent symptoms" can have various meanings.

Sometimes, it's the patient who is silent. Very few people ask questions. Deep down, they don't want to accept that they could be responsible for a potential change in their outcome. On the surface, that seems ridiculous; who wouldn't want a long life, one that has quality and vitality? Well, millions of people who end up with lifestyle illnesses, that's who—because taking responsibility for something requires us to change our mindset.

Some of you may be thinking, *That seems a little harsh*. I admit—it's a bold declaration to suggest that many do not want to take responsibility, but I am passionate about addressing questions until we get to the root cause of what's going on.

And if we have taken the time to identify that root cause, it grieves me if someone decides they do not want to make a couple of small changes to reverse it. That's the other form of silence—when the patient is aware, either through test results or some other indication, that they are headed down a dangerous path yet they still ignore the warning signs because it would force them to make a lifestyle adjustment to change course.

If I had the opportunity, for example, I would ask my father if he noticed a few things that seemed "off" and willingly chose not to explore them because he didn't want to know. Or did he get the tests and willingly choose not to make some lifestyle changes? I will never know because he's no longer here to ask.

Then, there is the third type of silence, the one we are most familiar with: "Well, I don't have any symptoms, so I must be in good health," which still amounts to not asking questions about their:

- Energy level
- Weight gain
- Stiff and achy joints
- Digestive problems

These are signs and symptoms of inflammation, which is the starting point of so many diseases. These little "whispers" are indicators that your body needs your help. Sure, a lot of things slow down or change as we age, but that doesn't mean we can't influence the outcome. I'm sure my father-in-law is stiff and sore, but he still runs. He doesn't accept or submit to that early-morning stiffness. It doesn't stop him from lacing up his shoes and getting out there.

Why is it important to look at these little issues now instead of five years from now? Because when we ignore the signs of aging, our aging accelerates. Today, you might experience a bit of stiffness that can be addressed. Tomorrow, however, you might experience a sudden episode that dramatically affects your life.

When that sudden episode happens is when someone usually comes to me for help. The conversation starts with me asking them, "When did you first notice this?"

"Well, you know, never. I've never had any problems."

"Never?"

"Well, you know, my back has been a little stiff and sore…."

In other words, they ignored the whispers until they became a roar. When your body roars, you can no longer restore things to how they were in the pre-whisper days.

The whispers are windows of opportunity. If you don't pay attention and make minor changes, it will speed up the process of degeneration.

If we knew the potential effect the whispers would have on our mobility and the things we want to do, we would likely pay far more attention to them. We don't make the association between pain and disability; we have a little pain, take something for that pain, and don't address the root cause of the problem.

Instead, we wait for some Big Thing to occur. We can't get out of bed. We can't put our socks on our feet. We can no longer swing a golf club. It was "sudden," and we can even pinpoint the day the Big Thing happened. Now we're motivated because the pain is taking things away; either they are routine things that are small yet significant, like the socks or getting out of bed on our own, or they are things we enjoy, like golfing or hiking.

Sometimes, by the time the Big Thing occurs, it will be too late. That was the case with my father.

I want to help you avoid that Big Thing, regardless of whether it's fatal, debilitating, or a persistent nuisance. The most difficult thing for me to observe is seeing someone in a post-Big Thing state and knowing they had a window of opportunity they chose not to take. Usually, they failed to connect the small whispers to a larger, deeper problem.

Think about it this way: If you were to visit the dentist and they noticed a spot on one of your back teeth that showed some signs of decay, what would you try first? Likely, being more diligent about brushing and flossing. Brushing and flossing will not eliminate the decay; the damage is already done, but it will help slow the process or prevent it from getting any worse.

By the same token, you can't totally reverse joint degeneration. But at the first signs of pain, you have an opportunity to make small changes today that can have a significant, long-term effect on your health. Wouldn't it be great to be an active seventy-five-year-old instead of a bedridden one?

Healthspan vs. Lifespan

Generally speaking, people are living longer thanks to technology, science, and medicine. If you had a heart attack today, the chances of you pulling through are far better than they were forty years ago. It's great that we live longer, but are we staying healthy as we age?

That is the concept behind the term healthspan: your ability level and health as you age. It's not just how long you live but how long you live disease-free with mobility and vitality.

Personally, I don't care as much about how long I live as I do about how well I live. I'm not interested in being in some nursing home, being fed my meals, and just being kept alive by certain medications or machines. I want to decide and define how I live my life.

Take This for That

Part of the problem is we have become a "take-this-for-that" society. For example, I could have said, "Well, my dad had heart disease, so I am going to take this medication," and fooled myself into thinking that was the solution. Most people don't think, *I'm thirty pounds overweight, so I better get my weight under control or pack a healthy lunch instead of wheeling through a drive-thru.*

Think about the last time you caught a virus; after about three days, if not sooner, you decide to hit the over-the-counter meds to make your life a bit less miserable. Or perhaps you ran a fever, your body's natural response to some type of invader.

Something has triggered your body, and your body says, "Something foreign is in here; let's fight it." The natural response of the body is to increase its temperature so you can better fight whatever is in there. Why should we allow the body to do what it's supposed to do? Because if we suppress the fever, we sustain it, and it will remain in our body longer.

Now, before you email me to tell me how dangerous that is, I'm holding up my hand to tell you there is a limit to this. I'm not suggesting a very high fever, like 105º F, should be "ridden out" instead of seeking medical attention. I am saying most fevers do not get that high, and as soon as we feel an inkling of one, we tend to reach for something too soon to knock it back down.

Pain is another one—we reach for an anti-inflammatory or some type of pain killer. I have patients who take it even before they play sports or exercise because they know they will be sore later. They do that instead of listening to their body telling them something is wrong. If you don't feel the pain, you could do even more damage.

Symptoms are a sign that something is wrong, so another part of the solution is getting to the root cause of the problem. That requires us to acknowledge the symptoms and, instead of just trying to alleviate them, use them to show us the real culprit. If inflammation is the overarching issue, we must adopt lifestyle habits that address it. Otherwise, the body can't self-heal and self-regulate.

If you are experiencing joint pain, lack of energy, poor digestion, or other symptoms, your body is already telling you something is wrong. We are so used to suppressing those signals and symptoms that we just keep adding more and more load without addressing the cause.

In fact, most people don't even know to ask the question, "What can I do to change this?" It hasn't occurred to them that they should play an active role in their own health. We ramble along, letting health hit us instead, but when it does, it's bad health (i.e., the Big Thing), and we immediately put ourselves in reactive mode. We reach for the closest thing we know, a pill or a prescription, to make it go away. We take this for that.

In many respects, it's the easy way out: "Mr. Jones, you're diabetic; you are always going to be diabetic. Here's a medication you have to take." Okay. Simple enough, right? But it's not a real solution.

A bit more brain power and proactivity is required to understand why we have Type 2 diabetes—to understand which foods create changes in blood sugar and which should be eliminated from the diet so the blood-sugar spikes stop occurring. It takes a few minutes longer—really, only a few—to grasp the bigger picture of what's happening than it does to pop a pill. But those few minutes can make a lifetime of difference.

This process is not about no longer trusting your doctor. In fact, many physicians and clinics are studying preventive medicine and rethinking their prescription processes. One physician here in Canada works exclusively with Type 2 diabetics, putting patients through nutritional protocols and fasting protocols, and they are seeing a lot of great results—many of their patients reduce or eliminate their medications.

However, we're too accustomed to letting someone else make decisions for our health. There is a big gap between an individual's understanding of what someone can do to make a difference in their health and letting someone else determine or dictate what they need to do (or take) to be healthy. It's all reactive. Take this, for that. Simple, but not a long-term solution.

Yes, There Is An Agricultural Component

Another part of the problem involves agricultural practices and food access. Today's farming practices and soil content are quite different from thirty years ago and dramatically different from one hundred years ago, all of which significantly affect the quality of our food. Studies have examined the vitamin and mineral content of foods today versus forty years ago, as well as the nutritional content of organic foods.

When you modernize wheat production, for example, what happens to the plant and its effect on blood sugar? I have European patients who are intolerant to wheat grown in North America, largely because glyphosate, a non-selective herbicide, is still used in North America. Glyphosate is no longer sprayed on European crops. Read Dr. William Davis's book *Wheat Belly* for a deeper understanding of wheat and its effect on our physiology.

More evidence is emerging that tags industrial seed oils as culprits that create inflammation. These oils have chemicals added to them and then are oxidized; they are highly reactive in the body.

They are also cheap. Soybean, corn, and canola oils (as well as other seed oils) are used in processed foods here in North America. If you look at the areas in the world where people live the longest and healthiest, they are not consuming industrial oils. These areas, known as the "Blue Zones," are known for different dietary and lifestyle habits. Part of their success lies in the absence of certain foods and ingredients—what they *don't* eat, which is highly processed foods, sugars, and these less healthy oils. In Greece and Italy, where a lot of people easily live into their nineties and hundreds, the consumption of olive oil is huge. They use healthy oils and healthy fats in most of their foods.

I would be remiss not to mention food access as another part of the problem. I'm not talking about starving nations and famine, though those are concerning. I'm talking about food deserts within North America and how they affect the health of those who live in those communities. These people literally lack access to good, whole food. It's a socioeconomic problem whose solution is outside this book's scope. I do think, however, it is important to raise awareness of the connection between certain groups of people more prone to certain types of disease and health conditions due to lack of healthy food access. Processed food is less expensive, typically has a longer shelf life, and ultimately, wreaks havoc on our healthcare system.

If you are reading this book, however, you likely have the means and the resources to make better choices.

Inflammation

Inflammation is at the crux of metabolic syndrome and the Big Four. When we look at cancer, heart disease and neurodegenerative diseases (like dementia and Alzheimer's), we know this inflammatory process is at the core of what starts to break down in the body.

How is inflammation created in the body? Poor lifestyle choices—lack of proper sleep, smoking, excessive alcohol, poor diet, and so on—produce an inflammatory environment. When your cells are inflamed, it creates a cascade effect on other cells in the body, causing changes throughout.

A good example is what happens in arteries. When the vessels are inflamed, they send inflammatory chemical messengers to circulate through the body, affecting different tissues; in cartilage, that will manifest symptoms of osteoarthritis; in the vessels, it manifests as cardiovascular disease and neurodegenerative disease. Your body does its best to repair these things, but the damage will continue as long as there is an inflammatory environment.

You can, however, decrease inflammation.

Of course, sometimes the damage is already done. It's happening silently while you are unaware; you feel okay, you didn't collapse in cardiac arrest after eating a cheeseburger, your job is really stressful, and you keep telling yourself it's temporary...until The Big Thing occurs. Maybe it starts in your knees and you shrug it off; a little stiffness is no big deal, right? You rub some cream on them or take an over-the-counter pain reliever and keep doing as you've always done. Until your hips ache, your hands ache, your back aches... you have this multi-level symptom that's affecting multiple joints, and then a doctor tells you you're full of arthritis.

So many patients come to me with these symptoms, thinking it's just a bad knee when, in fact, it's connected to so much more. In those cases, we have seen improvement by adding some simple supplements and avoiding certain foods that cause an inflammatory response in the body. The problem is if this cascade goes on month after month, year after year, the joints will already be swelling, affecting the patient's range of motion. Who wants to exercise if their body is already in pain? Not exercising creates another cascade because the patient isn't moving as much as they need to. The ripple effects, the cascading in each, are chaotic and explosive. How can we manage the damage?

Each Day Matters

Your health is a cumulative process, so each choice, each day, matters. I'm not talking about being perfect; imperfection is built right into the plan I will present in this book. We know habits matter—we can build good or bad habits.

When we talk about changing our habits, right away, people get stuck on what they will miss, or that they'll have to work out for an hour each day. They will no longer enjoy their favorite dessert, will have to starve instead of running through a drive-thru, or never eat cheese again. That's not at all what I'm suggesting.

Before we get into specifics, I challenge you right now to implement 80 percent of the habits we'll discuss in Part II to align with how your body is naturally meant to work.

If you miss a day of exercise, it's not a big deal.

If you attend a birthday celebration and you eat cake, it's not a big deal.

If you go on vacation and drink more than you typically do, it's not a big deal.

In other words, don't get hung up on the 10 or 20 percent that you are, for the most part, giving up. You can still enjoy what you want to enjoy, but you have to get focused on what you intend to do most of the time. What will be your 80 percent?

Before you get overwhelmed, remember even a little change can make a big difference.

But if we continue to assume that because we don't feel sick, we're okay, our society will continue to see a rise in the rate of chronic diseases. If it doesn't happen to you, it will happen to someone you care about.

The nice thing is we have a choice.

Every day you choose not to take action is another day that disease slowly wins. Every day you take personal responsibility for your health, you win.

And I'll say it again: It doesn't have to be complicated.

A few simple steps can keep you healthy forever.

CHAPTER 2

The Solution

Part of how I help patients solve their health issues is by using a framework that I call the "Blueprint for Health." (See the image below.) I have used it for twenty years in my practice, and it is as applicable today as when I first started using it to teach patients about their health. I'll cover some of its components in this chapter.

We can classify all of our different lifestyle stressors into three major categories: physical, chemical, and mental/emotional. Examples of physical stressors are accidents and injuries, body imbalances, and excessive sitting. Chemical stressors can usually be grouped into "too much" or "not enough" of something. An example of "too much" chemical stress would be added sugar or things like pesticides sprayed on our food. An example of "too little" would be things like vitamin or mineral deficiencies. Examples of mental/emotional stressors are easy to think of in today's environment: finances, work, relationships, and parenting are all things most of us deal with in some capacity, day in and day out. These stressors occur day by day, but how you handle those stressors will determine how much remains and accumulates in your body. Your body can tolerate a lot over time...but there is a breaking point where we often start to see some type of dysfunction, symptoms, or what we would call "dis-ease." So maybe not a full-fledged disease—yet—but things like pre-cancerous cells that are developing more rapidly, weight gain, lack of energy, rising blood pressure, or joints that are starting to "speak" to you more and more. The "dis-ease" is your body telling you something is wrong.

As you start this process, the secret is not so much about trying to take bad habits away; the secret is to add small, simple changes to your life.

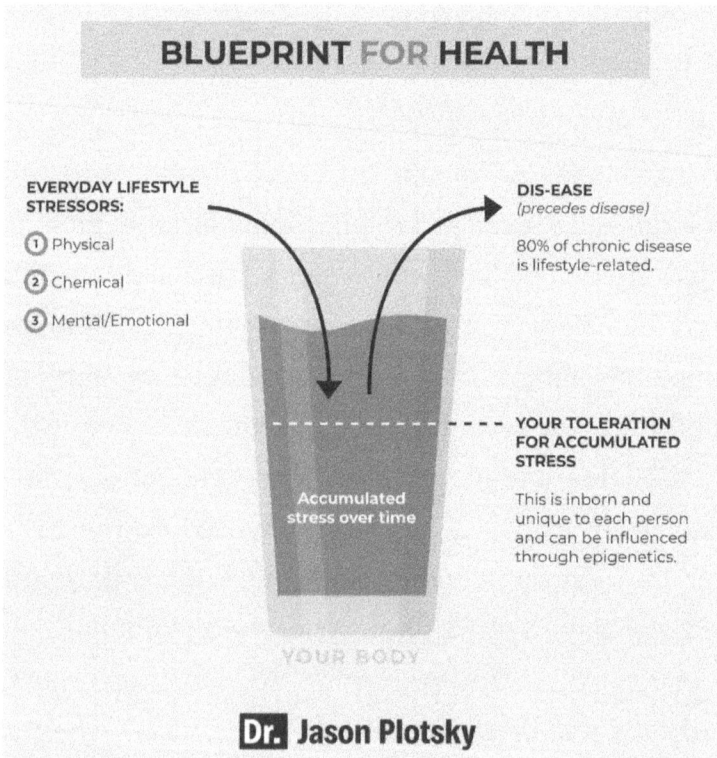

BLUEPRINT FOR HEALTH

EVERYDAY LIFESTYLE STRESSORS:

① Physical

② Chemical

③ Mental/Emotional

DIS-EASE
(precedes disease)

80% of chronic disease is lifestyle-related.

YOUR TOLERATION FOR ACCUMULATED STRESS

This is inborn and unique to each person and can be influenced through epigenetics.

Accumulated stress over time

YOUR BODY

Dr. Jason Plotsky

Addition, Not Subtraction

It is far easier for people to add in healthy behaviors than to take out negative behaviors. So, the answer isn't to change everything all at once; that's frustrating, tiresome, and quickly sets you up for failure. You want to stay healthy forever, not just for two weeks or a month. Our goal for you is to create a scenario that is sustainable.

Let's say you have five things you need to change; look at what you could add that will have the most profound effect on your health. What is the top priority, the one thing you can add that will not only improve your health but incentivize you to keep going because of its simplicity or benefit? Taking a step-by-step approach is best, starting with the easiest action item. For example, with many people who come into my clinic, water intake is the starting point. So, we may ask them to add a glass of water daily, which isn't difficult to do.

But They Have Meds for That

If you are diagnosed with a chronic condition before age sixty, it will affect your longevity. For example, if you are diagnosed with Type 2 diabetes, your lifespan will be shortened due to the other complicated factors that will often arise. If you receive a cancer diagnosis before the age of sixty, your chances of living past your mid-seventies decreases significantly.

Depending on your starting point, however, these effects can be reversed. We know that through lifestyle modifications, you can actually reverse Type 2 diabetes. Yes, some drugs can be used to manage it...but long-term, if lifestyle changes haven't occurred, your overall health is still jeopardized, and those drugs—insulin, Metformin, and so on—will not reverse the condition.

One of my clients, Joshua, was diagnosed with Type 2 in his sixties, and had been taking a couple of medications to manage it. Now in his seventies, he came to me because he was experiencing "foot-drop," the inability to control his foot.

The neurologist's report indicated that his most recent A1C, a ninety-day average of his blood sugar, registered at 7.7 percent. For perspective, a normal A1C is considered below 5.7 percent.

"You're on these two medications," I began, "and yet, your A1C is still really high." Usually, foot-drop is connected to the lower back, where the nerves control the leg. Typically, a disc herniation or something else exists that would affect the nerve's ability to control the lower leg. In Joshua's case, the MRI did not indicate that, so the neurologist concluded his muscular issue was due to his poorly controlled blood sugar. The best thing he could do would be to find a better way to manage his diabetes.

I asked Joshua about his eating habits, particularly meals. He was still eating quite a few carbohydrates in the morning— toast, cereal, things that are almost all carbohydrates. Lunch was usually a sandwich. His wife often made him muffins.

These people did not eat doughnuts all day; they understood the obvious carb culprits, like sweets and rich desserts.

But no one had educated them beyond sugary-sweet carbohydrates and their effect on Joshua's body and long-term health. In fact, they were told that these other carbs—the toast, muffins, and so on—were okay. He had his medications to keep him in check.

Except, they weren't keeping him in check.

"If this is happening to your leg, what's happening inside? We know the damage is taking place to your leg—but what about your arteries, heart, and brain?" Joshua and his wife had no idea that his blood sugar could eventually affect his heart or his cognitive function.

"Are you willing to make some changes?" I asked because I agreed with the neurologist—Joshua needed to get his blood sugar under control. Joshua and his wife were in complete agreement and willing to do what was necessary.

I handed them a small book I had written on the subject and told them to focus squarely on breakfast and lunch for now. "Don't worry about supper as much, and let's see what happens."

The following week, Joshua's blood sugar was under 7 percent. His wife came to the appointment armed with a list of questions. At that moment, I knew they were serious about changing things.

No one had ever explained Joshua's situation to them in a holistic way. He would have continued taking his diabetes medications, thinking they were taking care of things, and eating as he always had, unaware of the reverberating damage it was doing to his other systems. He had accepted that whether or not the medications were effective, he was stuck taking them for the rest of his life. He didn't understand the effect that his lifestyle could have.

We know that lifestyle choices have an effect on metabolic syndrome and The Big Four, and we know that The Big Four affect roughly 70 percent of North Americans; if we want to stay healthy as we age, then we have to make lifestyle changes to avoid The Big Four.

Allostatic Load

Simply put, allostatic load is the compounding effect of our lifestyle choices. When we look at the areas it can include, each one becomes a "load." For example, how many North Americans are carrying extra abdominal weight? That's a dangerous location to carry weight because this type of fat—visceral fat—accumulates and builds around our vital organs. Visceral fat is an allostatic load.

Another common problem is lack of sleep or proper rest. If you aren't getting enough restorative sleep, your body doesn't have a chance to recover from the day's stresses. That's another load.

Then there's the standard North American diet…processed foods, excess salts and sugars (hidden or unhidden), smothered, covered, fried. It's a chemical load on the body.

Lack of exercise and deficiencies (essential vitamins and minerals) are other loads.

Look, I live in the real world. If you saw me in a fast-food drive-thru with my kids after a particularly full day, I would likely shrug and tell you, "It happens." Some of these loads we could handle for a week or two because life happens, and it's not realistic to think we can eat perfectly all the time, exercise every single day, and get ample quality sleep every single night.

Over time, however, our lifestyle loads accumulate and compound. Your body, as intelligent as it is, is forced to adapt. It's always trying to counterbalance whatever stress you place on it to the best of its ability.

Therefore, this allostatic load gets heavier and heavier, month after month, year after year…and the breaking point occurs wherever your weak spot is. We know through genetics that some of us are prone to certain chronic diseases; some might be more prone to cancer, others more prone to Alzheimer's, and so on. Over time, this load will further these predispositions along, wherever your weak spots happen to be. In my case, for example, my weak spots are likely insulin resistance and cardiovascular concerns.

When you know where your weak spots are, you know where you need to put your focus. But there is more to the solution than strengthening your weak spots and lightening your allostatic load.

The Body's Wisdom

If we give our bodies the environment they need, they can respond—even if someone has Type 2 diabetes, even if they have already had one cardiovascular event or some other diagnosis. With the right opportunity, the body knows how to repair itself.

What governs the body's immune system? Or monitor the heart, the kidneys, the liver, or the brain? All of these are constantly under some type of control. Your body has this innate wisdom that allows it to already know what to do. As long as you protect your body from these different levels of interference, it can do what it's supposed to do.

I often say our bodies are smarter than science. They constantly monitor and measure to maintain a specific, balanced environment called homeostasis. The less allostatic load we put on the body, the better our chances of staying healthy.

Plug and Bail

Imagine you are on a small boat in the middle of the ocean when you drop something that tears a hole in the boat's floor. Now, water is rushing in fast, and you've got to find a way to save yourself. What are your options?

When I ask this question in my workshops, someone always responds immediately with, "Bail out the water!" That's true.

Then, after a couple of seconds, someone says, "You could plug the hole." That's also true.

Then I ask, "Which option will be more effective?"

You can bail, bail, and bail some more, but unless the hole is plugged, the water will continue to rush in. Bailing is similar to what we often do with our bodies. We use something to suppress the symptoms, but we never actually fix the problem at the source—we don't plug the hole, or stop that allostatic load.

Now, I realize it's not always quite so clear-cut. I live in the real world, remember? Sometimes, we don't know the source, don't recognize our role in the problem, and are in reactive mode instead of proactive mode. I see a lot of patients who are stressed; they have headaches, don't sleep well, and arrive at my practice with a host of stress-related conditions. I can't just say to them, "Okay, well, stop being stressed and a lot of these problems will go away." We can't just shut it off.

Plugging the hole, in this context, means locating and addressing the cause of the problem. It may not happen overnight, but to save yourself, it has to be your top priority. Once the hole is plugged, you have the chance to start bailing yourself out, which is where you can begin to apply healthier lifestyle habits.

What's your biggest stressor? What is the one thing creating the biggest allostatic load in your body right now? Remember, sometimes you can't get there right away, but you have to recognize it's there.

If the biggest thing is an inflammatory diet, you have to stop eating inflammatory foods. The miraculous thing about the body is you don't have to be perfect; even if you reduce that load by 50 percent, it gives your body a chance to respond. Not 100 percent—only 50. That's half your diet—not every speck of it.

I have seen, over and over, patients attempt some sort of hard reset, and it's quite admirable. If they can sustain it, I have seen dramatic repair happen in as little as two to four weeks. You will never hear me say this is the only way, however. Remember, I don't eat perfectly. Doing a hard reset and going cold-turkey-100 percent-all-in doesn't work for everyone. However, I've had patients who have suffered from miserable types of pain and dysfunction for years, and when we plug the hole—with better sleep, for example—and get them to where they can bail, I've seen their bodies responding in two or three months, many of them no longer taking the medications they were prescribed. They realize they may have been born with certain predispositions—but what they do to themselves actually puts them on a bad path. Once their pain is gone or they no longer experience headaches, they're ready to tackle more bailing.

For years, we thought our health was 100 percent based on whether someone had good or bad genes, but that's not always the case. For example, research shows there is a gene that relates to hangovers, but if you don't drink alcohol, it doesn't get expressed. Essentially, if you don't trigger the so-called "bad genes," they won't have the opportunity to express themselves. You side-step that health issue.

Many of us resign ourselves to genetics, and we just don't see the point in taking control or attempt to do so. While it's true you cannot change your genes, you do have power over them. For the vast majority of people, whether they side-step an issue or not is determined by their choices and environment.

My grandfather died at age fifty-five, and my father died at sixty-two. It seems evident I would have a weak spot for some type of cardiovascular event, but if I look at their lifestyles, it tells a different narrative. My father smoked until he was forty. He carried extra weight around his abdomen. He did not exercise, had insulin resistance, and in being self-employed, was responsible for several livelihoods besides his own. While he handled the stressors of his job fairly well, all of these environmental factors culminated in his allostatic load. Combine that with a predisposition for cardiovascular disease and you get a clearer picture of his "sudden" heart attack.

Your nutrition, exercise, and stress levels will all have a profound effect on your chances of developing something like Alzheimer's or cancer, or at least putting it off for a number of years.

Progress, Not Perfection

If we don't make that link between our lifestyle choices and our long-term health goals, we will not commit to doing better. When a patient tells me, "Yeah, I should probably exercise more and eat better," I already know their level of commitment will not sustain change. Those who turn their "shoulds" into "musts" are the people who can do hard things. They can make tough dietary changes, exercise when they don't feel like it, and get their stress under control.

Right now, you may be feeling like you're on the cusp. You're at a point where you are examining your lifestyle and thinking, "I want to live a long, healthy life. I'm committed to doing that. I want to hit my long-term health goals. I want to remain independent as I get older. I don't want any restrictions on my abilities to do hobbies, travel, and spend time with family."

If you are making that connection between your health and what you want out of life, then things are coming into focus, and what we will cover in Part II will make sense.

You can examine your lifestyle and determine your own starting point to implement very easy changes that make a lot of difference—I'll refer to this as Level One.

Over time, you may decide to take it to the next level, Level Two, so I'll cover how to take that next step.

To help you along, I'll remove confusion and the feeling of being overwhelmed regarding what to do. That way, no matter where you are on your health journey, you'll know what your next step will be.

It's important to me that we keep it simple because no matter your starting point, once you know it and what you need to focus on, you can make progress. And progress is what we are after—not perfection.

Now, it's human nature to want instant gratification. I will caution you: The strategy needed to reach optimal health takes patience. The longer the problem has been there, the longer it might take for the body to recover.

Here's a perspective that might help. I was at a lecture where renowned physician Dr. Deepak Chopra stated that 97 percent of the cells in your body will replace themselves in one year. That means that if you focus on certain areas of your life and lifestyle, most of your body will be completely different in one year. If we give your body the right tools and enough time, it will create an environment where healing can occur.

Emotional Leverage

We each have different types of emotional leverage. Do you want to see your children and grandchildren graduate from high school, take them on vacations, maybe even play a few games of basketball with them? Do you want to drive well into your eighties? Do you want to be able to travel anywhere, not just to places that allow wheelchairs? Heck, do you just want to be able to get on the floor and then get back up?

We underestimate the body's ability to recover in general, never considering all these little miracles that occur. Likewise, we underestimate the positive change that can be made through small tweaks. We think something like proper hydration or supplementation doesn't make much difference and downplay the potential effects it could have on our health. It's so much easier to dismiss options and never try them than to keep at it, right?

If you are serious about making these changes and creating a different outcome, you'll need to commit to doing the hard things. To succeed in doing those hard things, you'll need to tap into an emotional reason that gives you the leverage you'll need.

This emotionally charged reason is your *why*.

It will give you the power you need to keep up the small habits you'll be introducing into your life.

Sadly, most people don't know their *why*; therefore, they don't know what or who will keep them going—there's no real purpose for them.

We're going to make sure that's not you.

So, let's figure out your *why*.

Chapter 3

The Mindset

So far, you've read snippets of my life and quest to get and stay healthy. I couldn't have done all of it without the right mindset, and to show you just how important mindset is, I want to connect the dots and show you how I found my resolve.

I was a young husband and father, self-employed, and building my business. Life was good, but I realized my financial goals, my dreams, my "all" hinged on my ability to stay healthy. I'm glad I realized this early on in my adult life because, for me, good health makes it possible for me to reach my dreams. And I have big dreams.

In fact, anyone with dreams should understand that realizing those dreams will be affected by their health status, especially in their later years. In a strange way, what happened to my father and the reverberating effects it had on my family became a catalyst for me to say to myself, *Okay—everything hinges on my own health. I love what I do; I get so much satisfaction out of taking care of others…watching them heal, reach for their dreams, and attain their goals...but if I can't show up to work, I won't be able to experience that feeling of satisfaction, and nor will they.* Everything depends on my ability to get up every day and provide that service.

Now, at this point, you may be thinking, Well, that's easy for you. Health is your business. I sit at a desk all day—that's how I earn a living and pay my bills.

Health was not something that was given to me. In fact, genetically, the odds are stacked against me. So, I have had to develop good daily and weekly habits, too.

As a young adult, I thought I was already eating healthily. By then, I had graduated from the "teenager/stressed-out student" diet to what I considered a more adult, responsible diet. I had made an effort to cut out processed and fast foods, and I thought, *Well, I'm eating better than most people.*

Although health was on my radar, I wasn't eating as specifically as I needed to for my body to thrive. Understanding my genetics and how certain foods affected things in my bloodwork pushed me to take a closer look at my diet. Within three months of making a small change in my eating habits, my bloodwork changed for the better and I had more energy. Suddenly, I was empowered. *This is all in my hands,* I thought. *I am in control of this, not my genes.*

Once I made a simple change and saw its effect, I made another change. And another. At first, I had to tune in to take notice because, just like symptoms, the earliest signals are easy to overlook. But once I saw the powerful effect one small change could have on my life, once I saw the evidence, I was committed.

Finding Your **Why**

Knowing your *why* is important—it's the key to sustainable change.

Right now, you may be thinking, "Oh, that's easy. Why am I doing this? To get healthy." If that's your answer, then you haven't figured it out yet. You need to dig deep. *Really* deep.

Your *why* will commit you to your changes. It will sustain you on those days when you don't want to practice daily habits. When your drive wanes, your *why* will be your focal point to keep you on the right path. And the path is narrow—there will always be distractions and even some detours. But your *why*, centered on the horizon, will get you back on track and moving forward. Remember: Even if you stay on the path 80 percent of the time, you'll be so much healthier than you were when you first picked up this book.

If I don't help you discover your *why*, I can't help you link together your reasons for change. Then, when life happens—as it most assuredly will—you'll get lost in the weeds of "I'm too busy," "I feel fine; I don't need this," and "I'll just eat a salad every now and then, and I'm good." The excuses will come easier and easier because you haven't created enough leverage to actually change your habits.

Getting to your *why* requires an epiphany. Once it clicks, you know you're in it for life.

So, ask yourself, "What are my dreams? In twenty years, *what* do I want to be able to do, *who* do I want to be, and *where* do I want to be?" I'm guessing you didn't answer, "Bedridden."

I walk my clients through an exercise called The Seven Levels of Why. They are almost always surprised at how deeply I challenge them to go. A typical conversation might go like this:

"Mrs. Jones, what is your main goal for seeing me?"

"I want to lose thirty pounds."

"Tell me why you want to lose thirty pounds."

"I want to look better."

"Why do you wanna look better?"

"Well, I know if I look better, I will probably feel a little bit better about myself."

"Okay, great. Why is that important to you?"

We keep drilling down, deeper and deeper, to get to the core of what's going on. It usually takes me asking *why* about six or seven times for us to get there.

You may know *what* your goal is, but you also need to know *why* that goal is important to you. No one can come up with the reason for you.

Each person's reason for starting this journey will be different, and my role is to serve as the vehicle to help you discover what that reason is. If I can draw that out of you, then we'll have leverage and you'll have a much deeper, more focused understanding of why your goal is important to *you* — not to me or anyone else.

Maybe your *why* is quality time with your grandchildren, or a specific hobby or sport you enjoy. For others, like me, your *why* may be mission-focused — you have specific goals and a desire to do something purposeful.

I've included The Seven Levels of Why exercise below. Set aside at least twenty undistracted minutes to complete it. Walk through each level — don't skip any — and by the time you reach the final one, you will have discovered your *why*.

Without your real, authentic *why*, everything will remain a "should." I *should* stop this habit; I *should* pick up this habit. Shoulds don't provide enough leverage, and you need your *why* to turn that should into a *must*. When something becomes a must, you have enough leverage to sustain consistent action. Don't stop until you have that level of clarity.

The Seven Levels of Why

Pick your number one goal:

_____

Why is that important to you?

_____

_____

_____

Why?

_____

_____

_____

Why?

_____

_____

_____

Why?

_____

_____

_____

Why?

_____

_____

_____

Why?

_____

_____

_____

Why?

_____

_____

_____

Found your *why*? Good. Now we can get to another key part of crafting a mindset geared toward change: inspiration.

Inspiration vs. Motivation

Do you know the difference between inspiration and motivation? They're not the same.

I can motivate people externally for a period of time, but if they're not inspired, that motivation won't be sustained. Inspiration comes from the inside, from your core, and—like your *why*—it speaks to you in ways only you understand.

You may have a general idea of what you need to do to be healthy, and maybe even to avoid The Big Four. You get motivated, declare the "starting Monday!" battle cry, and do (or attempt) a three-week or thirty-day challenge. But the changes are short-lived. They didn't become part of your life, your routine. They didn't become automatic, like brushing your teeth or changing your clothes.

If you want ongoing and sustainable change, it all comes down to how you create the leverage that inspires you to do so. If your doctor tells you to quit smoking or cut down your sugar intake year after year and you haven't made a change, it's not that you lack the willpower—you're just not inspired. You haven't found your *why* yet.

When you're inspired, everything changes; the question goes from "Now what?" to "What next?" When you're inspired, you're in the right position to develop the right mindset to catapult you toward change.

Two things will help you work through this: patience and persistence. You don't want to burn out, after all! We'll talk more about pacing in Part II, but understand that all-or-nothing can burn you out. And frankly, no one is asking you to go from zero to sixty; we are talking about zero to one or, in some cases, zero to 0.5, even.

Setting Goals

When it comes to health goals, most people are too vague—they want to "lose weight," "exercise more," or "eat better." When setting health goals (or any goals), I'm a firm believer in the SMART method: Your goal should be something that is *specific, measurable, attainable*, and has a *realistic timeframe.*

Losing weight is an excellent example. It's not enough to say, "I want to lose weight." That is a valid goal, but it's too vague. How will you ever map out how to get there?

When someone comes to my practice and wants to lose some weight, I usually ask them to pick a number. Usually, they overestimate what they think they should lose or could lose. If they say anything over thirty pounds, I'll often cut it in half. So, if they say they want to lose forty pounds, I will counter with twenty. Why? Because while they were specific, and something like weight is measurable, forty pounds would take too long for someone who is just starting out—it's too far in the distance. Forty pounds can be a great long-term goal, but twenty is more easily attainable. The goal should fall within a realistic timeframe—twenty pounds in five months, for example.

In fact, if someone has struggled with weight, I might even pick a different metric, like waist size, to take their focus off the scale. People are very emotional about their weight, and if they put on a few pounds after trying to work on it, they get discouraged.

You always need to circle back to your *why*. It is essential to connect the dots between your health goals and the bigger purpose they fulfill so when you hit a roadblock, you don't completely derail. This is about progress, not perfection. When working toward your goals, you want to focus on positive progress and not just that micro-goal that hasn't been met... yet.

Now that you've found your *why*, which gave you your *must*, you're in it for the long haul. This isn't a quick fix, and it's important to take a breath and accept that. Any symptoms you are feeling, particularly those related to The Big Four, didn't just occur overnight—they've been building inside you for much longer. Accept that you're not going to turn everything around overnight, either. Lasting, sustainable change is not on a deadline; have patience with yourself and your body and take this one small step at a time.

There will be days when you get mentally fatigued and wonder, *What's the point?* This is where persistence and your *why* step in—when you don't feel like doing the things you need to, persistence and your *why* will help you stay connected to your goals. There are many days when I really don't feel like exercising, but when I connect to my *why*—something beyond myself—I remember that each day matters. Each step matters. Each change matters. Keep going.

No Willpower Required

Too often, we don't try because we think if we can't do something perfectly, there is no point in even trying. You doubt whether you can do it this time because you have tried so many times before. You think you have no willpower. But we humans default to the habits we have. Not happy with your health? Then let's look at how to better set you up for success.

Instead of relying on willpower, let's focus on something you often have control over—your *environment.* We want to shift your focus from relying on willpower to what you can control.

Let's say you want to make one change in your life—reduce your sugar intake. If you are a chocolate addict—maybe you keep a secret stash in your pantry—you can probably hold out for a couple of days. Then, life happens. You skip lunch, have a stressful day at work, frantically drive across town to make an appointment you'd forgotten about, and now having the chocolate feels more rewarding (or pacifying, or comforting) than not having it. If the chocolate is in your environment, odds are you're eating it. You need an environment that supports your decision; the fewer barriers you can create at this stage, the better.

At this point, you may feel vulnerable and uncertain that you can pull this off. (Don't worry; I know you can!) Don't let your past behaviors limit your thinking of what is possible. I've had many patients give up the "thing" by following the plan I'm laying out for you here. You can too.

I often tell clients they are "an average of whomever they hang out with." No one is suggesting you give up your friends and family, but consider whether they are supportive of your decision. It's one thing if you've told them and they still tempt you or say things like, "One time won't kill you"; it's another if you've privately chosen to change and know that time with them usually involves something that would derail you. If it's the former, you need to set some clear boundaries with them; if it's the latter, consider finding alternative ways to spend time with them, like going for a walk instead of going out to eat.

Developing the mindset that change doesn't need to be perfect, just consistent, can be calming. Remembering you are striving for progress instead of perfection can give you the confidence to keep going—or even just get started. Forget about past behaviors and willpower and focus on setting up your environment for success.

Change Your Identity

At some point, you will need to change how you see yourself in order to achieve and keep your health goals. This is another component of mindset: identity. Up until now, you may have seen yourself as a weak person with no willpower, someone who struggles with commitment, or some other negative self-identifier that sabotages who you are becoming. Do you currently see yourself as someone who can make a change for a couple of weeks, or someone who has healthy goals and ambitions? If you don't see yourself as a healthy person, you'll always go back to whatever you think you are.

Reaching a point where you identify as someone who can make long-term, healthy changes is key. I'm not talking about making a couple of changes and calling it done. Mindset cannot be overlooked. It will propel you to do the harder things for a longer period of time. Your health affects every aspect of your life—spiritual, financial, vocational, relational, and so on. You need to know where in your life you place the highest value.

Cue Your Why

If you link your health to how it influences your highest value, that also creates leverage. If you're an executive, for example, your vocation and finances might rank fairly high while your health might be farther down the list. If you connect that better health gives you more energy and more mental clarity to make sharper decisions, increase productivity, and so on, you will stay inspired to do the hard things. Linking your highest value with your long-term health is one of the biggest connections you need to make.

As you change your identity and move further into your health journey, you may also discover that your goals change… and your *why* might, too. In fact, you may learn you have more than one *why*! Usually, this is because you are reaching higher, broader, and deeper. Regardless, your *why* will remain a central driving force for your choices.

My initial *why* was for my family—not only to provide for them but to have more time with them. My *why* still includes them, of course, but it has reached beyond personal reasons— good health is my mission; helping others and serving them is my purpose. My health goals have extended to get this message out to as many people as possible.

And the bigger your goals, the more leverage you create. By writing this book, I am choosing to have more eyes on me than ever before; how well will my message be received, for example, if I take up smoking? My *why* includes a much larger accountability, and I have no intention of shrinking it.

But wait, you might be thinking. Didn't you say you hit a drive-thru sometimes? And if I ran into you in the grocery store, I might see some items in your basket that don't exactly jive with your message?

You're absolutely right. I don't always hit the mark of being my ultimate self every day, every hour, every minute. Because just like you, I am human. I still see patients full-time and have three very active boys. As I get closer and closer to whom I think I'm here to serve, however, I take those hiccups in stride. That broader audience still propels me forward and keeps me grounded. I can identify with their pain points and challenges, maybe not line-for-line, but there will always be parallels that keep me connected to them. We are all works in progress, and this journey is about progress—not perfection.

The Difference Between Knowing and Doing

A distinction exists between people who don't know what to do to get and stay healthy and those who do know and aren't doing it. Most of us fall into the latter category. We know we should eat "healthier," but we don't necessarily know what healthy is because new information is released all the time and we don't make it a point to stay current on this information. Others may not know their weak spots, genetically or otherwise, and they don't know their lifestyle will affect those weak spots. They might know they should exercise, but they don't necessarily know why—beyond looking good. They aren't aware of the other implications.

In my workshops, I give a crash course on how the body works, keeping it as simple as possible. It creates a deeper understanding for participants and provides them with another piece of leverage; once they understand how the body works, they are encouraged to take action. They realize they actually do have control and can make the changes they need to slow down, or even reverse, some of the effects of aging. Here is where the power of habits comes into play and sets you on your mission toward a healthy future.

CHAPTER 4

The Power of Habits

Jane, who was in her early forties, came to me for relief from severe headaches and back pain. As part of our assessment, I zoned in on specifics—her body's systems, other remedies she'd tried, and so on. With headaches, there is usually a long list of things to check off to narrow down the source. One of those things is diet.

"Well, I'm addicted to sugar," she replied. Admission is half the battle.

"What is it, exactly, that you're addicted to?"

"Oh my God, I can't live without Nibs," she said, pulling a small bag from her purse. "I eat a bag of these each day."

Looking at the half-eaten bag, I saw she was consuming 75 grams of sugar just from that indulgence. That didn't account for the sugar she was consuming in other foods.

"Okay, first, we need to set a goal of getting you under 15 grams of added sugar per day."

"I can't do that," Jane replied. "I cannot go without these."

"You don't have to," I explained. "Let's figure out how many Nibs equals 15 grams of sugar."

Jane took to this system pretty well. Each day, she'd take out the number of Nibs that equaled 15 grams of sugar and put the rest out of sight. Just like that, we were on our way to breaking her habit and making sustainable change.

For you, it may be chocolate almonds, chips, watching too much TV, or some other habit you recognize isn't great for your health...but you have no idea how to quit. You can't imagine yourself without it. You may even justify it: "I'm allowed to have one vice."

Maybe you have tried to quit, perhaps even cold turkey. Your intentions were good, you were resolute, but it all came crashing down in a matter of days. That's the problem with bad habits—they've been with you for a while, and most people can't stop overnight and be done.

Since you and I are not face-to-face, let me just let you know I'm not going to say, "You need to stop XYZ. Like, right now. This moment. Forever and ever." Whether that's eating sugar, smoking, drinking three beers at night, falling asleep in front of the television, eating when you're not hungry, or something else, you likely already know some of the things you do regularly that are not great for your overall health and longevity. If you are physically and mentally addicted to something, someone telling you to stop serves no purpose. You already know you should stop, but it all seems so...*final*.

In Jane's case, she wasn't willing to give up her habit completely, but she was willing to take control. Eventually, she arrived at a place where she could finally address her headaches and back pain. It's not always about quitting something as much as it is about dialing it back and managing it. If this resonates with you, you may need to cut down gradually or compromise with an 80/20 approach, like Jane.

However, for some people, it's easier to go all-in—100 percent—than to do it at 98 percent. Sometimes the very act of deciding to quit, cold turkey, removes the temptation and makes it easier to follow through. If you're someone who thrives on a total commitment, this may be the approach that works best for you.

Decide Which Approach Is Right for You

Whether you decide to cut back gradually or quit entirely, both approaches have their benefits. Here's a breakdown for each with tips for success no matter which camp you fall in.

Cold Turkey (100 percent commitment)

Why this works: This approach may feel extreme, but it can have a quick, noticeable positive impact on your body and your mindset. By completely eliminating the habit, you'll see whether the change makes a positive difference. It forces you to confront the issue head-on and can give you the clarity that you're fully committed to a new direction.

Tips:

- Identify the habit and commit to stopping it entirely.
- Set a firm date to start and prepare mentally to remove it without exceptions.

- Set your environment up for change—eliminate triggers or temptations as much as possible.
- Celebrate your success after a week or month of cold turkey to reinforce the change.

Gradual Reduction/Compromise (80/20)

Why this works: For some people, trying to quit all at once feels too overwhelming. Gradually cutting back or finding a compromise allows you to maintain some control without the all-or-nothing pressure. This way, you can still experience improvements in health while easing into a new routine.

Tips:

- Set a timeline to reduce the habit slowly, aiming for a manageable reduction each week.
- Track your progress by noting when and how much you engage with the habit.
- Replace parts of the habit with healthier alternatives—if you're cutting back on sugar, try healthier snacks like fruit or nuts.
- Reflect on how you feel with each reduction; some people find the habit naturally fades away when they give themselves room to adjust.

The cold turkey method might be right for you if you want a decisive break, but if you prefer to ease into change, the 80/20 approach could help. Either way, the key is to commit to the process, whether that means a sudden stop or a gradual transition.

Bad Habits vs. Addictions

I probably should draw some distinction here between an addiction and a bad habit because the process for escaping either will be different. Addictions get into your brain chemistry and neurological loops. When someone tells me they are addicted to sugar, it means sugar stimulates a chemical response in their brain's reward center. This response creates a sort of loop that compels the behavior to continue. Emotional triggers often amplify the craving, further activating the reward center and completing the loop. The cycle continues because their body physically feels some type of reward from their consumption.

A bad habit, on the other hand, doesn't create this same physiological scenario. While habits can also feel automatic, they don't involve the chemical dependency or compulsion we see in addiction. Habits are often tied to routines or cues but remain far more easily adjusted. You can coach people out of bad habits a lot easier than you can someone who has a bona-fide addiction. When someone is truly addicted, you can't expect them to do any sort of "two-week challenge," or quit cold turkey. Yes, I realize exceptions exist, but overcoming addiction typically requires a deeper, more intensive approach.

Here is where the *why* factors in.

If you don't connect with *why* you want to end an addiction or bad habit, it will be especially difficult to do so. Willpower can work for a period, but lasting success also depends on creating an environment that supports your goal. Using food addiction as an example, the culprit cannot be in your environment—not in your pantry, your refrigerator, your car, or your desk at work. Until you can discover your *why*, you won't find the strength to overcome it.

The difference between a *should* and a *must* applies here. If you haven't made that leap from a *should* to a *must*, then it's really just a good idea rather than something you're committed to changing. That shift is critical to creating the positive momentum needed to hit your health goal. Even if you attempt to quit, at some point, you will fail if your environment and mindset aren't set up properly.

The Environmental Impact

As you fine-tune your *why*, consider what will get in the way of you hitting your goal. The more obstacles there are, the less chance you have of hitting it. For example, if you have an exercise goal, consider questions like:

- What time of day do you have the most energy?
- When do you have a window of time?
- What exercise equipment do you have at home or close by?
- Do you have a gym in your apartment building?
- Do you have an inclement weather plan for exercising?

Let's apply those questions using a goal to walk briskly fifteen minutes each day. What time could you do that? If it's raining, snowing, or sleeting, how can you still accomplish it? Maybe you could walk the hall or stairs in your apartment building and not get completely off-track. Asking these questions is how you can craft a program that's almost foolproof and helps you succeed, no matter what.

Parents, especially, often have chaotic mornings. Trying to get lunches packed, kids off to school, and clear enough of the kitchen mess so it's not waiting for you when you come home…it's fair to say that mornings may not be the best time for you to exercise. You'll miss your chance more often than not, which doesn't help you develop a good habit.

Maybe you travel a lot for your job. How do you clear the obstacles of an inconsistent schedule, hotel rooms, packing, and travel days?

If you're making a food change, who does the grocery shopping? If you're not the grocery shopper in your family and you're trying to get rid of whatever it is—potato chips, chocolate—and your spouse or partner keeps bringing it into the house, your environment will have obstacles that force you to rely on willpower, and you can only rely on that for so long.

It's important to figure out what your obstacles are. Putting them on the table so you can really zero in on what is likely to get in the way is a huge part of setting up your environment.

When I help people develop good habits, I encourage them to keep changes small and incremental. For example, many people will declare, "I'm going to go to the gym one hour each day!" That works for about a week, and they feel good about themselves…until something gets in the way.

I coach people to initially think in terms of ten- or fifteen-minute windows and how to make really good use of them. Ten or fifteen minutes is better than nothing, and *some-thing* is always better than nothing...and certainly better than giving up altogether because you think you don't have the time. Then, as we build the habit of adding in small windows of exercise, we can progress to more.

You will achieve the most success in hitting your goals when you have the least number of obstacles. If you focus on your environment and try to remove as many obstacles as possible, it will increase your chances of success.

Compared to What?

When trying to make choices, sometimes you have to think in terms of, *compared to what?* Let's say you're not in the perfect environment to make a change; then ask yourself, "Perfect compared to what?" If you are attending an event or you're at a friend's house for dinner, and there is already a set menu that you have no control over, you simply try to make your best choice possible. We can't always control our environment, and that's just reality. Sometimes, you have to make choices in the realm of, *compared to what?*

There is another side to this—excuses. Here is where I normally ask a lot of questions because it's where clients can easily get derailed. I will have clients say, "I was doing okay, and then I went to my friend's house, and they were having cake. And I just don't have the willpower." Well, of course not—willpower is temporary, right? And if cake is being shared among friends, who wouldn't want to be a part of the fun?

Yes, this reveals weak spots, but remember—it's about progress, not perfection. It can't be all or nothing because so many of us don't have the perfect environment—we have kids or don't have the money or time.

If you can maintain good habits 80 percent of the time, that's progress. That's 80 to 90 percent of the results compared to what? Zero percent attempt. We have to get out of the all-or-nothing mindset; otherwise, we'll give up at the first sign of derailment.

In our living room, I keep several items to remind myself of the habits I work to maintain. My wife doesn't love it, but I know myself and my environment. I have my yoga mat, foam roller, blocks, and bands that I keep visible to remind me to do stretching and mobility exercises. If our family is watching baseball or a television show, I might take a few minutes during commercial breaks to get on the floor and do some stretches. I'm still there with my family, but I am doing something beneficial for my mobility. I recommend this for my mobility patients—keep your equipment close to where something else already happens. If you sit at a desk or watch television, take a few minutes to stretch or do some mobility work—no, it's not a forty-five-minute yoga class, but *compared to what?* Five to ten minutes of stretching is better than no minutes of stretching and losing your mobility in the process.

All Habits Have Power

How do habits factor into the success equation? First, understand that any habit, good or bad, has the power to influence your success.

Just as bad habits can accumulate negative effects over time and contribute to that allostatic load (see the previous chapter), good habits can accumulate positive ones. And it's possible to add a new healthy habit in as little as a few weeks.

Now, if we're able to link that new healthy habit to your *why*, over time, that healthy habit makes a huge difference. For example, if you were to add one supplement, like magnesium or fish oil to your daily routine, how would that benefit the cells in your body as they replicate and reproduce? Essentially, from a cellular level, you will become a new person a year later. The idea of adding one thing is great—but doing so consistently, over time, is what makes the difference. Doing something once isn't enough to make a difference.

This is the key to understanding the impact of bad habits, too. If you have a lot of healthy habits and you make an unhealthy choice one night at a restaurant or have birthday cake at a party, neither will determine your long-term health outcome.

By stringing together as many small, healthy habits as possible—again, in small increments, not all at once—it will, in time, stop being a conscious effort and become reflexive and no longer feel like work. It simply becomes part of you, part of your new identity.

While we covered this topic in the previous chapter, it's worth mentioning again: If you want to be a healthy person, you have to identify as a person with healthy habits.

How do you see yourself? Do you see yourself as someone with no willpower and the inability to control what goes into your mouth, or as a person who can't control their own time and schedule? Or do you see yourself as a healthy person who prioritizes all these little action steps, and knows it doesn't have to be perfect, just consistent?

As you stack your healthy habits, adding another and another over time, an amazing, optimized health outcome occurs. The cumulative effects of drinking more water, adding a stretch, walking ten minutes, and taking a quality supplement can all make a tremendous change in your body. Most people quit too soon. Apply the patience and persistence we discussed in Chapter 3 and accept that even though the results aren't necessarily immediate, they can be optimal over time.

Good or bad, your habits will determine your outcome.

Accountability

You've likely picked up on my insistence that this journey is about progress, not perfection, and hopefully, you've also realized I live in the real world and enjoy a piece of birthday cake now and then. If you spend most of your time on "detour," changes will have little to no effect because they haven't had enough consistency to accumulate. When I think about the workshops, programs, and courses I have conducted, those who experienced optimal success consistently made the neural connection between their *why* and the results they wanted, and they added a good habit or eliminated a bad habit as a result. They went through their Seven Levels of Why, they know how it all connects, and they have someone who helps keep them accountable. They might see me once a month, but they see their accountability partner more often.

You can do the same. For example, if you're trying to incorporate walking into your routine, you might have a walking buddy who checks in or holds you to your walking schedule. This is particularly helpful on days when it might be tempting to stay in bed. Then you won't feel like you're just letting yourself down; you are letting another person down.

I recommend finding an accountability partner who is firm and supportive. What I mean by that is someone who will hold you to task but not mentally beat you up about it. On days when you feel weak or tempted, a good accountability partner will help you unpack those feelings and remind you of your *why*. You can reach out to them when you're struggling.

If you find yourself spiraling into self-shaming, caught in a cycle of *Why can't I do this? Why do I always fail?*, an accountability partner is especially helpful. An accountability partner, group, or coach can help you mentally declutter and shift your focus back to why you are doing it in the first place.

Identity Congruence

I encourage my clients to think about their current identity and the identity they want to have in twenty years (aka, their future self). They might say, "Well, I really like to play golf," or something like that.

"Do you see yourself playing golf in twenty years?"

"Well, in twenty years, I'll be [whatever age]. I hope so."

"But your mobility isn't good now. Do you think you'll be able to hit that goal if you don't make any changes?"

"Hmm…probably not."

"What do you need to do on a daily or weekly basis to be able to still play golf in twenty years?"

Most people know what that looks like, but they don't often connect that it is the path to getting there.

Earlier, we discussed the idea of changing your identity and identifying as a healthy person with healthy habits. That was in the immediate, the present. Now I'm asking you to make that identity congruent with your Future Self, the one who is ten, fifteen, or twenty years older.

Personally, I know I want to play golf, coach baseball, or play catch with future grandkids; I want to travel with my wife and not have any restrictions about my ability to walk, hike, or climb. I also understand if that's what I want in my future, what I am doing today, tomorrow, each day, week, and month will determine the outcome.

If I'm going to accomplish that and more, I would have to be at a healthy weight. I would have to exercise daily, stretch, take any required supplements, and sleep well. My life should contain a lot of joy and happiness, with good social networks. I would need to have my stress under control. Every day I ask myself, *What do I need to start doing today to create that outcome that I'm looking for?*

Sometimes, our present self doesn't factor our future self into our goals, and that often creates two different identities.

So, we have to take that future self and coordinate it with our present self to craft the plan that will achieve and sustain the lifestyle level we wish to maintain.

Let's say you see ten healthy habits that your future self adopts, but you only have one healthy habit in the present. You already know you'll have to incorporate nine more, but you don't have to have all nine in place by tomorrow. You add them over time; let them accumulate one by one and stack them until they are congruent with the person who is doing what you want to be doing in ten, fifteen, or twenty years.

What is your biggest future health goal? If your mind just went completely blank, know that you must start to see yourself in the present and the future, and understand that what you are doing daily or weekly will determine whether you reach those goals.

Many times, we are ensnared in this trap of bad habits with the mental block of "Someday, I'll..." or "I really should...":

- Lose the weight
- Quit scrolling on my phone at night
- Stop drinking soft drinks
- Eliminate processed foods

And so on. We continue doing the same thing over and over, but we're unhappy, and deep down, we know we are incongruent. Many don't care, don't know where to start, or they start and fail, so they're frustrated or overwhelmed.

Let me reassure you: That's normal.

Let me also reassure you there is a way out of this cycle.

There will be days when you are frustrated or overwhelmed. Congruence isn't a linear path—there are zigs and zags. You won't always see what's around the corner, but you have to maintain that clear vision of what your future self looks like, feels like, and is doing. It's not enough to say, "I want to be healthy," because you have to define what that looks like to you and how it will affect your dreams.

Rewiring Your Brain and The Power of Anchoring

Neuroplasticity refers to the brain's ability to learn new things. When it comes to habits, this ability is what we are trying to tap into. If I have a patient who is in the habit of reaching for a cookie immediately after finishing dinner, we have to rewire their brain so this action doesn't take place—either they no longer want the cookie, or they reach for a better choice instead.

We also have to sustain the change—that's where that magic window of 21-30 days comes into play. Usually, if you can do a thing consistently for that period of time, you have improved your chances of turning it into a habit.

This 21-30-day window doesn't create permanent change for everyone, however. For some people to break an old habit or create a healthy new one and sustain it, they need to rewire their brain.

Each time we perform a new healthy behavior, we make healthy neural connections that over time will help us incorporate that new behavior into our lives. And when we connect a new habit to something we already do, called *anchoring*, that also rewires the brain so we can create new, better habits.

Every day, I try to help patients find ways they can use anchoring in their day-to-day lives. If I'm working with a patient on their back mobility, for example, I don't show them a stretching exercise and tell them to figure out how to incorporate it into their day. Instead, I might ask, "What is something that you do every morning without fail?"

They might reply, "I brush my teeth every morning," or "I make coffee," or "I read the news...."

"Great," I respond. "Now, immediately after you do that, and each time you do that, do this stretch. It will take you less than three minutes."

Nearly 100 percent of the time, they will smile and say, "Okay, that seems simple enough."

Then I follow up with, "And I will have you report back to me how many days you did it the next time I see you."

Usually, their smile tweaks just a bit, because now I have placed a measure of accountability in there. It gets them thinking. By anchoring the new behavior to an older, established behavior, and then reporting back to me, they keep better track of what they are doing and how often.

That is another reason an accountability buddy is a good idea. You could just as easily text someone or take a photo of a meal and send it to an accountability partner—that accountability can be huge for helping to rewire your brain.

The accountability increases your chances of getting it done, and anchoring the new habit to the current habit increases your chances of incorporating it into your lifestyle.

The Roadmap to Breaking Bad Habits

From a psychological point of view, it's much easier to add something in than it is to take something away. That's why we start this process of change with the first five habits we need to add to our lifestyle.

Developing good habits is a great starting point, but eventually, you will need to look at your existing habits and determine if you can modify or eliminate those that do not serve your health. Awareness is key, but many people are unaware of what their habits are, good or bad, until they take inventory.

I won't tell you to write down everything you do on a certain day. Rather, focus on the habit in question (or the habit you already know needs to change). Whether the change involves food, movement, sleep, or something else, you need an awareness of your baseline and what you're currently doing.

Let's use sleep as an example. You already know you're not getting enough sleep, but you can't pinpoint what's going on. To get started, you might write down everything you do at least an hour before you go to bed, log what time(s) you wake up, and do this each day for a week.

This sort of exercise gives you conscious awareness of what you're doing while focusing on one bad habit at a time; otherwise, there is a good chance you will never break the bad habits. It's important to link the bad habit to something painful or something that won't be attained, like a goal, if you don't break it. Then—because you want your current self to be in congruence with your future self—inventory and awareness let you consider the impact the bad habit will have on your future self if you allow it to continue. Use the questions below to help you get started.

- What is the habit I want to change?
- If I keep up this habit for the next twenty years, what will it cost me? (think health, relationships, finances, etc.)
- If I change this one habit, what would that create for me or give me?
- What would that feel like?

You must be honest with yourself here. Until we know how bad something actually is, and we don't dismiss it, we'll never kick the habit. I can't tell you how often I hear, "Oh yeah, I don't really eat that badly," and see people dismiss taking the inventory. Or they skew the behavior—either by underreporting or "behaving" for the week—so the "report" looks good to their accountability partner. That takes a lot more energy than just getting to the truth, right? Be honest with yourself.

As humans, we downplay how frequently we do certain behaviors, and then we also downplay what the potential effects of continuing that behavior would be. Unless we bring that to light, we can't truly understand how bad something is, which means we don't know how hard it will be to change. If you recall from the last chapter, when someone has a bad habit, it will take a significant amount of leverage to make a change—in other words, pulling out all the stops.

Look back at the questions above. Did you sort of smile at the idea that a bad habit could cost you your life? You might have wondered if I was being melodramatic, but consider whether there is something today you've done that, if you repeat each day for the next ten to twenty years, might shorten your life. Shorten the time you have with your loved ones. Shorten the time you have to accomplish your dreams, reach your career goals, and check items off your bucket list...shorten it to the point where you might not have twenty years to continue the bad habit. What happens to your spouse, your children, your grandchildren, your dog, your home, and all the things you worked for if you're not around?

Let's get real for a second here: What sort of reverberating impact would this have?

Until we hit a pain point, most people do not realize their health will affect other people or other things. The pain of discipline will outweigh the pain of regret every day, so pick your hard. At some point, we have to get real, take inventory of what we are doing, and acknowledge it's probably destroying our bodies on some level. And if you have any sense of your future self and future goals, there is only one way out: changing something.

Change is difficult, but remind yourself, *Sometimes it's harder to think about change than to actually do it.* If nothing changes, nothing changes.

Final Thoughts on the Power of Habits

Remember Jane, the client who was addicted to eating Nibs every day? She's still a rockstar. She's crushing it at the grocery store, taking walk breaks at work, and is 100 percent off her Nibs now. It didn't happen overnight. She had to build it up, one day at a time, until she went a full week without one. Once she got going, she just rolled with it. Her confidence grew. As she learned more and more about herself, she realized 100 percent was best for her.

I have other clients who shoot for 80–90 percent. Some can even sustain 98 percent; they just need to know they still have that option should they choose to take that detour. Every day, I am blown away by someone who has figured out how to connect the dots and has been able to make very powerful changes—things they didn't even think were possible a few months before.

What story are you repeating to yourself about your habits? That they don't matter? That you'll start on Monday, next month, after the holidays, next year? That it's not that bad? Everyone else is doing it (or everyone else is doing worse)? That you're weak and spiraling into a pit of guilt and shame?

Take a moment to sit with your *why*. Every time you keep that promise to yourself, it will help you build the self-esteem and confidence to keep going. The kept promises will start to accumulate, and you'll amaze yourself because deep in your heart, you'll know that this time, you will succeed.

Most of us generally take our health for granted. If we don't start taking a serious account of what we do every day, seven out of ten of us will end up being another statistic of chronic disease. Where does health fit into your values? You need to know the answer before moving on to Part Two. To determine your answer, look at the wheel and shade in the areas according to your personal value system. For example, if you would rate your health an 8 out of 10, then shade it up to the 8. If you would rate it a 6 out of 10, then shade it to a 6. Repeat with all the values so you can get a visual of where your health is in relationship to all of the other aspects of your life. For physical surroundings think of things like your home, car, clothes, etc.

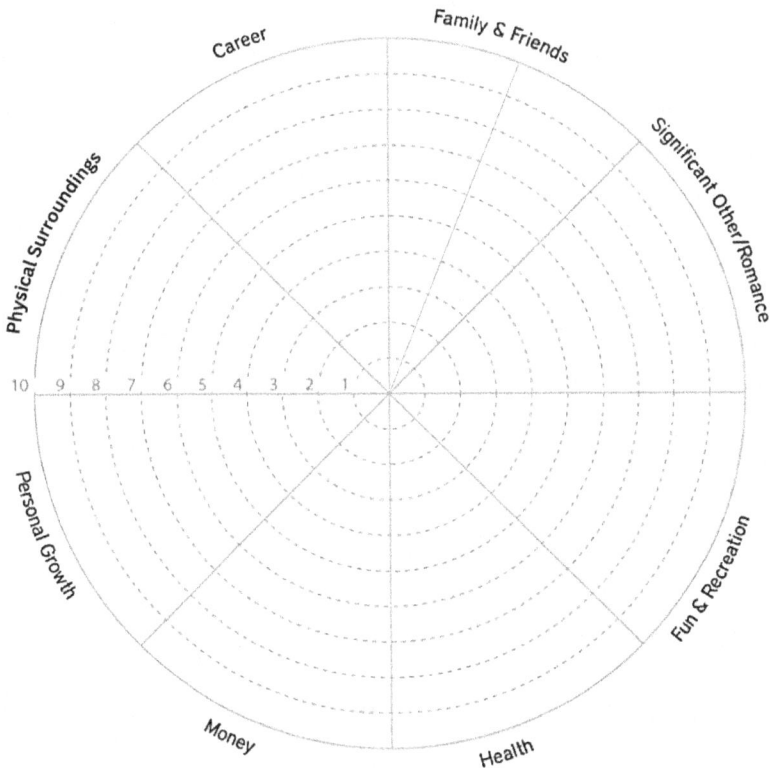

You can also get an extra copy of it in the resources section by downloading the QR code:

If you don't have a clear understanding of where health fits into your values, then the incorporation of different types of habits will fall by the wayside at some point. If you haven't secured a solid mindset, one that powers you through, it's because you don't know *why* you're doing it. Revisit these five essential questions and write down your answers:

What's your one-year goal?

_____

_____

What is your twenty-year health goal?

_____

_____

How would you describe your best future self?

_____

_____

Where does health fall on your values system?

_____

_____

What is the number-one habit you need to change right now?

_____

_____

Make sure you can answer those five questions before you turn the page. If it helps keep you accountable, enlist a friend to do it with you and message each other when you are done.

You need to be certain of your long-term goal, short-term goal, and dreams, and be certain that health ranks high on your values scale in order to achieve those goals and dreams. When you know the answers to those five questions, you will have the leverage and the power to make any change you set your mind to.

Ready when you are.

PART II:

The Six Pillars of Good Health

Most people have never done the kind of deep work we're doing in this book, the kind that teaches you the extent of how you limit yourself and your thinking. Just because you haven't attained your health goals before, or even considered what your health goals are, doesn't mean you can't do it now.

My mission is to help others achieve optimal health. To do this, I developed a simple plan of actionable steps that are sustainable, buildable, and yield results. The key driver will always be your *why*. At the end of Part I, I asked you to complete five questions before turning the page. You've done your homework, correct? You know your *why* and how it will affect your health today, tomorrow, next month, next year...and its effect on others.

Part II introduces the pillars, which are six areas in each person's life that encompass our habits, good or bad.

The Six Pillars of Good Health are:

1. Movement
2. Mobility
3. Sleep
4. Supplementation
5. Food
6. Stress Management

While we'll examine each pillar in the subsequent chapters, I always encourage people to look deeply at the areas where they feel particularly vulnerable. For example, we'll spend some time examining sleep, but you may want to go even further and expand your knowledge by reading another book devoted to sleep. You can also do this for nutrition, mobility, and so on. As humans, we may be inclined to think if we "fix" that one problem—whether it's sleep, nutrition, movement, mobility, supplements, or stress management—we have fixed them all. But that's not really the case.

Another angle we need to take involves taking an honest look at your fitness level. My coaching clients take an assessment to help determine whether they are a beginner (Level One) or an intermediate (Level Two) when it comes to health.

To break it down more clearly:

- **Level One:** If you have been truly sedentary and have never considered nutrition or supplements beyond marketing gimmicks (i.e., "fat-free," "all-natural," and so on), put yourself at Level One.

- **Level Two:** If you have a regular walking schedule or have made an effort to cut down on processed foods, you may be a Level Two.

There is also a Level Three (think elite athletes), but I won't be addressing them here.

This book is for those who have tried to get healthier, given up, and tried again, and for those of you who want to do the work to address their daily aches and pains (besides popping an anti-inflammatory and calling it a day).

I'll talk more about Level One and Level Two in the following chapters and give you specifics for how you can approach improving each pillar based on your level.

Each pillar is important, and each person will prioritize the pillars differently. But even if you read this book and only take into account that each area will, eventually, require you to take inventory, you will still have a firm grasp on what you need to do to optimize your health and longevity.

And when your desire for change supersedes your desire for comfort, change will happen.

CHAPTER 5

Pillar One: Movement

Barbara was suffering from neck pain, headaches, and a generally "blah" feeling about herself. She had no motivation to exercise because anytime she tried, it just seemed to make things worse.

I needed about a month to get a read on whether Barbara could be self-motivated to make some changes. She wasn't going to do that unless she felt better. If I could take away even some of her pain, she might keep going.

"Would you be willing to commit to 150 minutes of exercise each week?" I asked.

"That sounds like a lot. I'm not sure I can commit to something like that," she replied.

"Okay, let's break this up into ten-minute walks, maybe two each day. Could you fit in one in the morning and another in the evening?"

"I can try," she said, smiling.

A few weeks later, walks became part of Barbara's routine. She would walk for ten minutes in the morning before work and take her second ten-minute walk either during her lunch break or after she arrived home in the evening. Eventually, she started taking longer walks on the weekends because she had more time to do so.

After a couple of months, I asked Barbara how it was going. "How do you feel after you walk?"

"I have so much more energy!" she exclaimed. "I can focus better when I'm at work, and I'm sleeping better, too!"

Movement is one of the most underrated and powerful tools we can use to move the needle in all aspects of our health. It's usually the first issue I address because it's easy to focus on, and if you're a Level One like Barbara, it's easy to apply that basic metric of 150 minutes of exercise a week.

Movement also affects more than our physical health. Many people suffer from mental health issues. While movement won't resolve the mental health issues that need constant medication, for those who suffer from depression and anxiety, movement works wonders.

When you move your body, it stimulates the brain. In Barbara's case, she was more productive at work. Over time, she also started sleeping better. In the meantime, I was applying chiropractic care to address her pain, so she was in less and less physical pain, too.

Walking produced a real domino effect in terms of tackling other health-related issues that were within Barbara's control.

Within that second month, she was making better food choices. This is common because exercise often becomes a catalyst for other changes.

By the third month, Barbara had a chat with her doctor about not taking her antidepressants anymore. She was sleeping better, feeling better, had more energy, and was in less pain. Her doctor agreed and tapered her off. By the fourth month, Barbara was completely off her medications and highly functional.

Barbara's success wasn't quick, but she just needed that spark to connect her *why* to her habit, and she was off!

Our Bodies, By Design

Our genes today are almost identical to how they were ten thousand years ago.

Some research estimates that they would have moved approximately thirteen kilometers a day—approximately eight miles. That's a lot of ground to cover, and a lot of movement, largely to secure enough food to eat. By comparison, today we mostly sit—not just at our jobs, but in our commute, watching television, and even our hobbies—most of us sit maybe eight hours or more each day. Eventually, chronic issues arise, like joint pain or weakening muscles because our bodies are not in use. The longer you sit, for example, the more your muscles shorten to accommodate. Then, you try to pick up something heavy or attempt something else your body isn't used to doing, and ouch. You blow out your back or shoulder.

When you consider what our bodies were designed to do and what we're doing now, a massive gap exists in our lifestyle—not our genes. We don't even have to go back ten thousand years; we could go back one hundred, maybe one hundred and fifty years, and the gap is already there. They had fewer cars on the road then so people had to walk everywhere—work, school, market, church. When you look at pictures from 100 to 150 years ago, very few people are overweight.

From there, fast-forward to the 1960s. It was common for families to have a car, but most were not two-car families. People still walked or rode a bicycle to run errands, visit friends, and so on. We were not in front of computers or playing games on our phones. We were outside working in the yard and our daily activities were just that—active and requiring physical strength and endurance.

Now look at where we were just forty years ago. As a kid during that time, I lived across the street from a park. Unless it was pouring rain, we played in that park every day after school, even through the winter. (I grew up in Edmonton, Alberta; if you look on a map, it's pretty far north, and it was freaking cold!) We slew dragons, saved the world as superheroes, staged our own Olympic games, or kicked around a ball. We'd play for a few hours until one of our parents got home from work. Then we'd retreat to our respective homes for supper. Not until I reached my teens did video games start to hit the market, and I had a couple of friends who stopped playing outside and started playing more video games. Barriers existed to getting those games then; you had to have a system and the cartridges or you had to rent them.

Today, it doesn't even occur to my kids to go out to play— my kids have no concept of what it means and won't go unless I kick them outside. They'll ask me, "Play what?" while we have a trampoline and a basketball net and there's a batting cage next to our house....

When you consider that kids are being paid to play video games—and some make decent money—it's tough to argue they should play outside for the sake of their health. But experts are saying that sitting is the new smoking, and when it comes down to it, our bodies are designed for movement.

If we're not moving as we age, we reach a point where we don't want to move anymore. And our bodies accommodate— to their detriment.

The Brain Connection

Movement stimulates the brain. If we want to keep our brains healthy—remember neurodegenerative disease is one of the Big Four—regular exercise plays a large role.

As you exercise, you increase the blood flow to your brain. This helps keep the tissue healthy, and it helps fire neurons, too. Essentially, you create more neural activity when you move.

As we become less active, our aging process speeds up; the brain is less active, we move less, we have less oxygen going into our tissues, and we have less circulation. Here is where that visual picture of your future self becomes very important. If you see yourself as an active person twenty or thirty years from now, you have to be moving now in order to be that person. Your brain requires stimulation—and movement triggers the kind of stimulation you can't get sitting in front of a computer.

Ten Minutes Can Change Everything

At this point, you might be thinking, "I don't have time to exercise for an hour each day."

No one is asking you to. Often I don't have an hour to spend at the gym either.

If you are brand new to exercise, then start with the minimum effective dose of exercise; for most people, that's about ten minutes. That may be a daily total for you if you consider yourself to be at Level One; if you're a Level Two, you may find two or three opportunities to incorporate ten minutes of exercise each day.

In either case, make it a micro-goal to build to approximately twenty minutes total each day, whether that's two, ten-minute intervals or the full twenty minutes all at once.

Your next question might be about levels of intensity. Are we talking about ten minutes of leisurely walking to the store, or high-impact, sweaty exercise?

This goes back to your individual fitness level. If you are a self-proclaimed couch potato, it's probably not a good idea to attempt a six-minute mile. So, walk a twenty-minute mile or ten-minute half-mile. Something is always better than nothing, and you will always have ways to expand and improve your exercise.

Right now, your target is 150 minutes per week—that's the amount the Cancer Society, Heart and Stroke Foundation, American Diabetes Association, Diabetes Canada, and Alzheimer's Society all agree helps you decrease your odds of chronic disease—specifically, the Big Four.

Is Movement the Same as Activity?

I always ask my patients if they exercise. Occasionally, some reply, "No, but I'm really active."

What exactly does active mean? Many of us wear fitness trackers. I can track my steps through the day; the nature of my job earns me anywhere from 10,000 to 13,000 steps a day. If I only do that, however, will I hit my health goals?

Our fitness levels naturally decline with age, so simply being active isn't enough. If you want to be able to lift your grandkids up or hike a mountain at seventy, you must start pushing yourself now.

Easy Ways to Work Movement Into Your Day

Pick one day over the weekend—Sunday is usually a good day for this—and review the week to come. Where are your appointments? Which days are you driving the carpool? Who has activities this week? Finally—where are your pockets of ten-minute or twenty-minute intervals?

Some days you will have more time, and some days you will have less. Look for ten-minute windows where you can add a little easy exercise like:

- A short yoga sequence

- A basic core routine
- A circuit of air squats, planks, and pushups
- Marching in place

If mornings are chaotic—cooking breakfast, making lunches, driving children to school, work, running in six different directions at any moment—then morning is not the time for you to look for these pockets. If you take twenty minutes to watch the news, however, maybe you do have time. Move your stationary bike into the TV room or take a walk while listening to the news. Instead of carving out extra time, find a way to incorporate movement into something you're already doing.

Yes, taking stairs or parking farther away helps—but ten minutes is the minimum to be effective, particularly for neurological benefit.

Levels of Movement

When it comes to being intentional about movement, certain thresholds help us gauge whether it's time to level up. Beginners (Level One): incorporate those minimum ten-minute intervals doing what you enjoy—walking, swimming, yoga. Shoot for a minimum of 8,000 steps per day—this can decrease all causes of mortality by about 40 percent.

If you fall into Level Two (intermediate), strive for at least 10,000 steps each day, seven days a week. At this level you should also focus on building and maintaining strength. That doesn't mean you have to join a gym or buy a lot of expensive equipment; it can be done in many different ways, including budget-friendly resistance bands, dumbbells, and even pushups or chin-ups. Depending on how hard you train, strength can improve with one to three sessions per week. Start slowly and work your way up. But remember, you can over train.

When you're ready to push yourself a little more, here's what that could look like for each level:

Level One: Aim for 8,000 steps per day and push for 20-30 minutes of exercise per day that leaves you out of breath.

Level Two: If you're lifting weights, try adding variety to your lifting and getting in basic pushing, pulling, and hinging movements. Incorporate squats, lunges, rotational and core work. If you're running or jogging, try sprints running uphill, or rucking (walking with a weighted vest).

Too Busy or Too Tired?

More often than not, clients tell me they are too tired or too busy to find the time for movement. The irony is exercise provides energy; but for some people, the thought of exercising is tiring.

Remember what I said back in Part One: Thinking about change is often harder than change itself. When we are tired, we can't see ourselves exercising—the thought of it is just exhausting. Fair enough. The actual physiology of it, however, will improve our energy, especially if we find something we like to do. Then it becomes a question of *when* we can do it.

Which brings me to the other complaint I hear: I'm too busy to exercise and really don't have time. My response is always the same: This is not about figuring out the perfect time to start; starting is the perfect time.

In both scenarios, I walk them through a battery of questions:

- How badly do you want to be healthy?
- Where in your daily life do you have ten minutes? (Because, as Tony Robbins said, "If you don't have ten minutes, you don't have a life.")
- If you don't have ten minutes for your health right now, where do you think your health is going to go in ten or twenty years?

If you're struggling to get started, don't forget to connect to your *why* and envision a version of yourself who can do the things you want to be able to do. A future you who golfs, hikes, does yoga, or swims. Even a future you who does activities not directly associated with exercise, like traveling or playing with grandchildren, requires two things: joint mobility and muscle health. You have to work on both to have both.

If you value your health highly, you'll find the ten minutes. If you don't, you'll find excuses. Then, if you make excuses long enough, your body will start to whisper to you....and if you ignore the whispers long enough, eventually, it'll scream.

Need an extra nudge? Enlist a walking buddy or accountability partner. Find someone who is either more motivated than you or more disciplined than you, and then piggyback on their influence.

Another question I'm often asked (usually by someone who doesn't want to start exercising) is: Is there ever too much exercise? The answer is yes. According to Ben Greenfield (expert trainer), this number is usually more than 400 minutes per week—it over-oxidizes your body. That's why marathon runners sometimes drop dead from a heart attack. It's not very common, but it does happen.

Injury is a more common issue related to too much exercise; in most cases, someone is doing high-intensity exercise that their body isn't conditioned to do. Everyone is different, but everyone still needs time for rest and recovery. I strategically have a day or two of what I call "active-rest" days, usually the day after my high-intensity training. My active-rest days may include a restorative yoga session, a longer stretch day, or a leisurely walk with my dog. I'm typically not lifting weights or exerting myself too much. I'm still active those days; I'm just not pushing myself or trying to set any new personal records.

Other Objections

If, as you've been reading, you've started a mental checklist of all the reasons you can't start, let me tell you this:

You can't afford *not* to work out.

Every day, I take care of people who wish they'd started sooner. You have an opportunity now to move your body and try to get to the next level.

What are you waiting for?

Many times, someone will tell me they can't afford to work out; gym memberships are expensive, they can't afford the equipment, and so on. Once again, I start them with walking because most people have a pair of shoes that are comfortable enough to walk in.

If they need more than walking, any number of online videos can be used for a home workout or yoga session (my friend Sarah has an amazing, inexpensive online platform called Angel Fish Yoga). A few weights and some resistance bands can be purchased for less than a hundred dollars.

Are you someone who says, "I just can't get up that early to work out"? Then you need to discover your natural rhythm. If morning workouts don't work for you, are there other times during the day or evening when you are energetic? Even if it's only for ten minutes here and there, maybe even while you're sitting at your desk.

Now, in some cases, you may not have control of your schedule. I still encourage you to look for windows of time you didn't know existed. You may need to squeeze in ten or twenty minutes during your lunch hour or find fifteen minutes in the afternoon or immediately after work. Make it a priority to locate those windows and pockets of time. They are there, I promise.

What if you have to go home for your children and to make supper? Evenings may be your only window, and I strongly recommend you take advantage of the time immediately following supper.

There is always a window somewhere; maybe you will have to wake up fifteen minutes earlier or rearrange some of your workday, but you do have two or three pockets of ten minutes a day, and they should be dedicated to movement.

Book It, Then Mix It Up

Schedule these ten-minute windows of exercise. Put them in your calendar and treat them just like any other appointment or meeting. Why is it important to have these on your schedule? Because if it's not scheduled, other things will creep into that space. That is especially true when trying to create a new habit, so take it as seriously as other meetings or appointments. It also gives you back some control over your schedule.

When it comes to specific types of exercise, mix it up a bit. My wife ran cross-country during her university years, so it's very easy for her to default to running. Running is an excellent sport—it's healthy and definitely buildable in terms of goal-setting. The problem arises when running—or any singular activity—becomes your only exercise. It's easy to skip when conditions aren't optimal; you may get bored with it. Also, you work the same muscles and joints, over and over again. To minimize wear and tear on your body and your joints, keep a variety of activities and exercises in rotation. All of your joints need to be put through the right range of motion, so there is no one "perfect" exercise (yes, that includes swimming).

Different types of exercise provide different benefits, and you want to create as much brain activity, blood flow, circulation, and oxygenation of your tissues as you can. In terms of longevity, having a certain amount of both strength and mobility is imperative, so keeping as much strength and muscle tone as possible is key. That's how you'll be able to do the hobbies and activities you want to do in ten, twenty, or thirty years.

Ultimately, what we're trying to do is build a body that has the ability to adapt. A variety of exercise types puts your body through different ranges of motion, different types of stress, and different types of loads on the muscles.

Time to Start Moving

If you're a Level One, moving your body daily should be your goal. Figure something out that you like to do that helps build strength and muscle health. Get those 8,000 steps in.

If you're a Level Two and already moving your body consistently, keep it up. Continue to find ways to challenge yourself and stay focused.

No matter your level, set a goal that stretches what you think you are capable of. Hitting your goals could mean the difference between being active as you age and being unable to do the things you hoped to do.

CHAPTER 6

Pillar Two: Mobility

John was a runner, and really fit. At thirty-three, he was also experiencing lower and upper back problems, which didn't make sense, given his physical fitness level. I decided to put him through the entire battery of assessments. Somewhere, something had been overlooked.

"Let's check mobility," I said, casually. "Go ahead and touch your toes."

John got as far as his knees before he grunted...and stopped.

"Are you stiff?" I asked. "Is your back stiff?"

"No," he replied. "That's as far as I can go."

I was puzzled. A guy who ran 10ks and half-marathons on a regular basis was unable to touch his toes?

"Okay, have a seat," I instructed. "Let's try a seated toe touch." That was even worse. My mind was blown.

In the previous chapter, I noted the difference between movement and mobility. To underscore this difference, you could be active all day, but if you don't have mobility in your joints and other parts of your body, you probably won't be able to hit certain activity goals in the future. John is a great example of someone whose activity was one-dimensional; he'd taken up running to lose weight, but he had never incorporated any other sort of exercise or movement to keep his joints and other muscles limber.

It was a wake-up call for John. Right then, he realized that while running has tremendous benefits, he couldn't expect to be fit, healthy, and strong if it was his only outlet. John had mobility deficiencies in his upper back and legs. He worked in IT, so he was also in front of a computer all day. Running didn't fix this for him.

In many of the chronic cases I see, the part of the dysfunction is away from the site of pain; you could have an old ankle sprain that screws up your knee or your hip, or old whiplash that affects your whole alignment. John needed to work specifically on his hamstrings and hip flexors. I showed him various stretches and exercises, explaining he had a lot of work to do. He could not expect to be able to touch his toes in two weeks or anything like that. Thankfully, he was motivated.

Many of the mobility issues I see come from sitting all day. I have had school-age children in my clinic who cannot do a half-squat because their back is so stiff from sitting—in class, on the bus, for lunch, on their phones. They're not even sitting with their backs upright; it's horrendous. Even with my own kids, I will say, "I can't believe you're sitting like that," but their bodies have accommodated it to a point that it's now "natural" for them.

Then, they attend university where there will be more sitting, more studying while sitting, to hopefully graduate and land a job where there will be even more sitting. Sitting is chronic, it's vicious, and it's landed most of us in a lot of pain, suffering from different types of dysfunctions that are actually fairly simple to resolve—if we are willing to put in the work instead of popping an over-the-counter pain med.

Mobility Hygiene

Dentists encourage us to practice good dental hygiene for a reason—the benefits go a long way in saving us money, protecting our health, and, frankly, making us enjoyable to be around. Part of my mission is to practice preventative measures before something becomes a problem, so I also like to help clients with various hygienic practices.

Mobility hygiene involves identifying weaker spots in our body and working on them before they start to hurt. If you took the quiz and figured out some parts are weaker than others, but nothing came up as a mobility issue, why would you want to wait until you have one? Anyone who has an active goal, whether to work longer, raise their children, or hike the Grand Canyon, requires physical health—including mobility.

Recently, a client in her mid-forties was trying my no-sugar challenge. We were discussing the ups and downs she had experienced. "Okay, let's take a step back," I said. "What is your long-term goal? Where do you want to be in twenty years? Thirty years?"

"Alive," she replied flatly.

"That goal sucks," I responded.

Interestingly, my office sits beside a hockey rink and an assisted living facility. Pointing, I said, "You have two choices. In twenty years, you could be over there skating, or you can be over there where someone wipes your butt because you can no longer do it yourself."

Then I said again, "Now, what do you want to be able to do in twenty years?"

"All the things I'm doing now," she replied. "I want to be able to walk, go to the gym, go for a swim."

I explained that if she wanted to swim in twenty years, she would have to have good shoulder mobility. Whatever movements we want to do in ten, twenty, or thirty years, we have to be able to perform now. If we can't, we need to start working on it. When it comes to mobility and movement, we're really in a "use it or lose it" situation.

Many clients come in complaining of hip pain. Maybe they even had it x-rayed a few years back, and it wasn't bad then, but the pain has increased. Now, they can't even put on their socks. The joint is completely worn out. If you have the money and time, you can see a surgeon—but why wait for it to get to that point?

When you are in miserable pain, it changes your mental health. We have to be careful about taking high levels of over-the-counter and prescription medications, like non-steroidal anti-inflammatory drugs because they can damage the lining of the stomach and have other serious side effects.

Exercise offers one of the most immediate and long-term benefits for health. If you want to live a long and healthy life, you have to exercise a certain amount each week. If you don't take care of your mobility, in time, you won't be able to exercise or even do mundane things, much less the things you enjoy. Mobility protects the hobbies and activities we like to do, so we need to do what we can to protect our mobility.

Think about the joints in your body—your shoulders, hips, fingers, elbows, knees, and so on. Think about your neck and spine. If any of those are stiff, you do not have full mobility, and therefore, you cannot optimize your movement. Using golf to illustrate this:

- If you can't get your shoulders over ninety degrees, you won't have a good golf swing.
- If you can't rotate your spine, you will struggle with a backswing or a follow-through.
- If your knees are worn out, you'll have to ride in a cart or struggle to walk.

Mobility is really about protecting what you want to continue being able to do, and there's more to it than simply having a good range of motion.

Mobility Outliers

I've emphasized flexibility in joints and muscles quite a bit in this chapter, but other areas to consider are your posture, grip strength, and balance. These also deteriorate as we age so they need our attention.

If you have bad posture and experience headaches, your body may be telling you that you have an issue. Poor body alignment affects our shoulders, pelvis, rib cage, and so on. Many of these offsets come from old injuries where the body adjusted to protect itself and keep going. In some cases, when the head and neck deviate from normal alignment, it's basically like a bowling ball on a stick. The rest of the body tries to balance the head, and eventually, things get pulled out of place from trying to compensate. Often, if I can get someone's head balanced, the rest of the body follows. While chiropractic has many approaches, this is my approach. I won't go into it too much here, but you can read more about it on my clinic website: www.NovaSpinalCare.ca.

In most cases, when someone's alignment improves, their mobility improves. As mobility improves, dysfunction reduces, and pain decreases.

Posture

When sitting, your ear should line up with your shoulder; for every inch it goes forward, the head's weight doubles the stress to the spine. Think about people who sit slumped in front of computers all day (we have the term "tech neck" for a reason!). Many of these people suffer from headaches originating in the neck. Because the head acts as a massive lever, the neck muscles must compensate, work hard, or tense up when the head shifts out of alignment.

If these distortions aren't addressed, they can become permanent.

This poor posture and misalignment also affect how well you take in oxygen because your breathing is affected. And if your oxygen intake isn't optimal, what does that do to the cells in your body?

Unless you're in outer space, your body is always under the force of Earth's gravitational pull, whether you're sleeping, lying down, or upright. How your body is aligned and where your head is in relationship to the rest of your spine becomes very important.

Correcting your posture — literally and figuratively — takes a weight off your shoulders!

Grip strength and balance are other mobility outliers — huge ones, in terms of aging. Recent studies have concluded that both are key predictors for longevity; a lack of stability and proprioception (the ability to sense our body parts' position, movement, and actions) lead to falls, which lead to things like hip fractures, which lead to things like accelerated decline. If someone over the age of seventy is hospitalized with a broken hip and they've lost mobility, they usually do not live much longer. Part of the strategy to combat this is to keep walking, yes, but also to work on deficiencies like balance and strength.

Wait a minute, you might be thinking. I thought something was better than nothing.

Yes, something is better than nothing. If you've developed a good habit of walking, then it's time to level up. That's the only way you'll hit those goals of swimming with your grandchildren or traveling without restrictions. If you lose your grip strength, how well will you cast a line? Or swing a golf club? Or control the steering wheel of your vehicle? Make a plan so you don't lose those skills and abilities—make a plan using your *why*.

Connecting the Dots

By now, I hope you are making the long-term and short-term connections that exist in how the body functions, particularly with regard to mobility. How we sit, for example, wouldn't seem to factor into our shoulder mobility, into how we reach above our head, yet it does. When we connect something that's important physiologically, we are more inclined to make changes.

Let's take some time now to rate your own mobility. Visit the online assessment on YouTube by clicking on the following QR code:

Whether you experienced any pain or not while doing this assessment, these are basic mobility patterns we should be able to do. If you struggled with some of these, let me assure you that all is not lost. At the same time, we need to examine your goal and possibly reset your expectations. There is always room for improvement, but depending on the extent of your inability, it will be more difficult to regain full mobility.

Protect Your Body so It Can Heal

The body has a tremendous ability to heal, and it will do the best it can with what it has to work with, so if we have great joint spacing in the spine and the discs are all healthy, someone who is simply "jammed up" will likely make a full recovery so long as they are willing to do the work. On the other hand, if someone comes in and they have severe spinal degeneration (which is the worst), they hurt in every direction, can barely lie down, and make noise when they sit or stand, they will probably never recover to 100 percent, but there is plenty of room for improvement. By putting your body through ranges of motion, you are doing something healthy for the body and for the brain.

Remember in the last chapter when we talked about how movement isn't just good for your heart but also good for your brain? Your brain is also always perceiving your joints in space; in fact, that's a good chunk of your brain activity. It is always asking, "Is this appropriate?" and trying to make sure everything is where it is supposed to be.

The more we move our joints, the better the fluid nourishes the cartilage around the joints and improves blood flow. All those things can slow down the wear-and-tear process. Even if your goal is not to get to perfect, just practicing your range of motion will improve your ability to act, react, and be aware of your body and the space around it.

You may not become a ballerina, but as you practice that single-leg stance with your eyes closed, you will form those neural networks that make your response faster and more sure-footed.

Reciprocal Inhibition

If I had to pick the three areas of the body that should get the most attention, they would be your spine, hips, and shoulders. When we're walking, standing, and moving, our muscles are working in balance; and if we sit for short periods of time—anywhere from ten to fifty minutes with standing and moving in between—it's not a big deal. There won't be a lot of issues in all the surrounding tissues for the hip.

Over time, your muscles can tighten and shorten, causing reciprocal weakness in the opposing muscle group. For example, during a bicep curl, the bicep contracts while the tricep relaxes. In the hip joints, constantly shortened muscles prevent others, like the glutes, from firing properly, causing weakness. This often results in lower back pain or tight hips, affecting your ability to squat, bend, and lift.

Not everyone with back pain has shortened hip flexors and weak glutes, but it is common among my patients. Because the hip joint is so central to the body, when it's not functioning well, it has a ripple effect on other body parts, particularly the spine.

Once you pinpoint which body parts need the most attention, can you devote ten minutes per day, or even one day per week, to working on them? It doesn't need to be overwhelming, but simple movements—like stretching or standing after every fifty minutes of sitting, or using resistance bands while watching television—can help you get out of dysfunction.

Use the above screening to determine which parts of your mobility could use the most work and watch the following video on YouTube for a demonstration of some mobility exercises.

There Is Always Something You Can Do

I hear this all the time when I'm conducting a new patient intake: "Well, you know, my mom had bad knees, too," or "My dad struggled with this as well." When it comes to mobility, how large of a role does genetics play versus the environment?

It's true some genetic connections exist to inflammatory conditions or being prone to inflammatory issues in certain areas of the body…but that doesn't mean you're destined for inflammation. Generally speaking, your inflammatory status plays a major role in your mobility and pain, but the idea, "It's old age, and the doctor already said there's nothing I can do about it," is ridiculous. While X-rays may be helpful to reveal the amount of degeneration in a joint, they don't necessarily define the outcome or the cause of the pain. There is plenty you can do to work on mobility and strength instead of popping a new prescription while waiting on a new artificial hip.

A few simple habits can bring down your inflammation and, by default, reduce your pain—including if you suffer from arthritis. Start by drinking more water—if you're not currently drinking water, commit to one glass per day. If you are drinking water, add one glass per day. The next question to consider is: Are there any supplements you could take to naturally reduce your inflammation? We'll take a deeper dive into this in Chapter 8, but many supplements specifically address joint pain.

Check your posture. I've already mentioned how poor posture can give you headaches. For more information on how posture affects your body, visit https://idealspine.com/understanding-the-role-of-the-cervical-spine-in-forward-head-posture/.

Arthritis and joint pain are not a life sentence. Don't let someone else normalize them for you. Yes, you may have some wear and tear on certain joints in your body, but there is always something you can do to improve your own health.

Mobility is the difference between being alive and having a life. If you want to be self-sufficient as you age, you have to think a lot about what you're doing daily or weekly with your body to ensure you will be. You can't bike, swim, play golf, or even pick up your grandchildren if your mobility is limited or, worse yet, lost. What you do today matters with regard to what you'll be able to do in the future. If you can't touch your toes, how do you expect to lift your grandchildren?

Working on things like hamstrings and hip flexors can go a long way toward alleviating lower back issues, even if you are an athletic person. Remember John, from the beginning of this chapter? At thirty-three, he started to understand he couldn't just go for a run and call it a day on his mobility. This guy could run a half-marathon without the traditional training, yet he could not touch his toes. So, he started spending a few minutes stretching after a run to make sure he wasn't recreating those tightness patterns.

You might be thinking you'll just wait for the surgical solution. Surgery always has risks and potential complications. People assume surgery will fix all orthopedic issues, but we should try all conservative measures first.

When we think about all these little strategies, particularly if we can hit peak performance, athletes and everyday people who have good mobility will always have the edge. Each pillar affects the others, and the relationship is often reciprocal. For example, if your joints don't hurt, you're likely to get a better night's sleep, and quality sleep gives the body time to do the necessary repair work to help alleviate pain. Too often, mobility is a massive blind spot for many active people who don't recognize its contributions to their overall physical health.

CHAPTER 7

Pillar Three: Sleep

Our pillars of health are deeply interconnected. An easy example is the connection between the stress our nervous system endures and our sleep.

My client Ann was forty and having neck issues. Many people initially come to see me for help with some physical pain, and Ann was no different; she had two kids, chronic neck pain, and trouble sleeping. She'd stay awake for hours at night, unable to unwind her brain. Her doctor had prescribed her sleep medication, but Ann didn't like taking it because it really knocked her out and made her groggy when she woke up. With two small children to manage, that wasn't what she wanted her mornings to look like. As a consequence, she would take the prescription maybe once per week.

We went through a checklist of everything Ann was doing before bed and what she felt was making it difficult for her to sleep. Most people can endure pain for short periods, but Ann's neck pain was ruining her sleep. Eventually, we settled on her trying a more supportive pillow and seeing whether that helped.

After a month of working together, Ann found it easier to get to sleep. It wasn't perfect, but by month two, she had nights where she slept through the night without the help of medication.

That added energy had a domino effect on the quality of Ann's life. She was more productive at work, and her ability to take care of her kids escalated; she had more patience with them and genuinely enjoyed parenting again.

Ann initially came to see me because of pain. Ultimately, addressing the larger problem of her sleep quality allowed her to make other changes that affected how much better she felt during the day.

Another client, Stephanie, was a shift nurse. She would work two days and two nights on, then four off—a demanding routine for anyone, but more so for a nurse in her sixties. Stephanie came to see me to address some back, neck, and hip issues that were giving her pain. As we discussed her health history, I asked how well she slept at night.

"Oh," she said, "I usually wake up at two or four, and then I can't get back to sleep."

She would try, of course, but she'd never succeed. Instead, she accepted it as her status quo. It became her pattern. She'd read books in the middle of the night for a few hours, occasionally dozing off. Her shift work had messed up her circadian rhythm.

This situation is sometimes common for younger patients who are on their phones all day and night or for people who watch intense movies or television shows before bed. Stephanie, however, didn't fit that mold.

Instead, we found she was too wound up at night. When she came to the office for her appointments, we worked on calming exercises; I showed her some breathing exercises and meditative techniques to slow her mind down before she tried to sleep.

With those small changes in her sleep routine, Stephanie began to see results. By the second month, she was starting to sleep through the night. This wouldn't happen every night; sometimes, she would still wake up early, but that shift was enough for her to notice major changes in other areas of her life. She felt much better throughout the day, and her cognitive ability massively improved.

Many people just accept that they can't sleep; maybe they are shift workers like Stephanie, busy mothers like Ann, or just accept that they are light sleepers. But a lack of quality sleep affects so many health parameters that it's worth investing the time to fix sleep issues. Who doesn't love feeling refreshed and ready to tackle the day?

It's common to struggle with turning your brain off before bed. Many people have racing thoughts that prevent them from going to sleep right away, especially if they go right from work mode to sleep. While there are things we can do in the office to help with this, sleep hygiene techniques, as we'll discuss shortly, can make a real difference. But first, let's understand why and how the body sleeps.

Parasympathetic and Sympathetic Nervous Systems

We have two parts of the autonomic nervous system: the sympathetic and the parasympathetic. They must stay in balance; spending too much time in the sympathetic state can make us feel stressed and overtaxed, affecting our mental wellbeing and ability to fall and stay asleep.

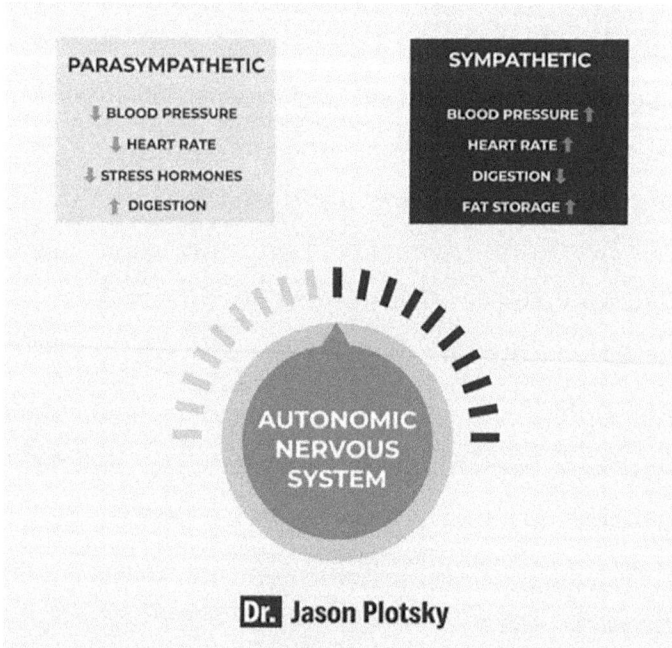

The parasympathetic nervous system is the rest and digest system. We want to spend most of our time there, in a calm state. The sympathetic nervous system, on the other hand, manages our fight-or-flight response. It allows us to take quick, decisive action and think clearly and instinctively in moments of crisis. It's good that we have both systems, but spending too much time in the sympathetic nervous system, or putting ourselves in situations where we need to be constantly alert or are often worried, wears us down.

Each system sets off a different neurotransmitter cascade. That means if you're in fight-or-flight mode, you secrete certain chemicals and hormones in your body to keep you alert, to help you feel less pain, and other things. However, when that system gets out of whack, it can tell the body to be alert at times when it really shouldn't be, like at two in the morning.

Circadian Rhythm

We were meant to wake and sleep with the sun. When camping away from city lights, your body naturally syncs with the sun's patterns. Our circadian rhythm, triggered by less sunlight, cues melatonin secretion for sleep. Depending on your chronotype (more on this later), you might wake earlier or sleep later, but generally, we follow the sun.

Different chemicals wake us up, but modern lifestyles disrupt this rhythm. Moving north with limited winter sunlight or even small shifts like Daylight Savings can mess up our sleep.

Other types of light can also affect our sleep. Red light is getting a lot of attention right now because of its many different health benefits, including mimicking parts of a sunrise. I have a red light at the clinic and use a red light at home. It makes me feel very alert when I use it in the morning. On the flip side is blue light, which also stimulates the brain and has gotten a lot of press for keeping people up late at night.

Blue light blocking glasses are becoming increasingly popular to aid with sleep hygiene. Some people are fanatical about it: they wear blue-light glasses, keep all their lights dark at night-time, and stick to a strict sleep schedule.

Sleep as a Health Practice

In the last few years, sleep has been connected to many other aspects of health. When someone tells us they're struggling to lose weight, we often ask what their nutrition and exercise habits look like. We rarely ask how they're sleeping.

Without enough sleep, our cravings increase, and we have more difficulty breaking down sugar. Yet we don't really think about this when we think of weight loss. We think of having energy or not, not realizing that sleep is vital to whether or not we have that energy.

It's easiest to see the effects of quality sleep on people when they're deprived of it. Studies show that when people are deprived of sleep, even in the short term, it affects their insulin responses and how their bodies process food. Satiety hormones, the hormones that tell you when you're full and that it's okay to stop eating, get messed up after just one night of not enough sleep.

To emphasize sleep's significant benefits for diet management, we need to consider its influence on two key hormones that regulate eating: ghrelin and leptin. Ghrelin is the hormone for hunger. Leptin is the hormone for satiety. Leptin, in particular, is affected by sleep deprivation. Studies show that even if you eat exactly the same foods in sleep-deprived and non-sleep-deprived states, your body will have less leptin circulating through it. You'll feel less satisfied and be prone to overeat. In this study, not only did the sleep-deprived subjects eat more calories, but they also gravitated toward more carbohydrates.

It may be a roundabout way of looking at it, but if someone says they're having trouble losing weight, their sleep may matter more than they think. It's part of a whole cycle, yet it's often not even in the weight-loss picture.

Certainly, when people talk about optimizing their health, they're willing to talk about sleep. Yet sleep is absent from discussions about Type 2 diabetes management, where lessening cravings and normalizing an insulin response would be incredibly useful.

Mood and how you feel throughout the day is determined so much by sleep; without enough sleep, people struggle and don't have the energy for the things they want to do. Mothers especially benefit from better sleep hygiene. In the early months of motherhood, it's easy for everything to get thrown out of sync: the baby wakes up at odd times in the night, and sometimes when you're up, you're up. However, even after the kids are sleeping through the night, sometimes mothers still struggle to sleep well. They're still in that sympathetic response state, too alert to get restful sleep because their brains have been trained to wake up at any noise.

A bad night of sleep affects the entire next day, and with the coping mechanisms that follow—drinking too much coffee, making poor food choices, skipping a workout—it becomes difficult to reach our goals. If we don't prioritize sleep, those coping mechanisms can become a bad pattern. Sleep has to be something we look at as a serious tool. People who don't sleep well don't even know what the body is capable of until they start resting deeply.

Getting restful sleep, on the other hand, sets us up for success in the day ahead by mitigating daily stressors. If you knew you could hand your body the tools it needed to unwind from a crazy day and make the next day great, wouldn't you use them?

Quality vs. Quantity

What should we be most concerned about—how much sleep we're getting or how good the quality of that sleep is?

My answer is quality. Deep, restful sleep does more for your ability to rebound after stress than lying in bed and tossing and turning.

Many people go through life pushing, pushing, and pushing themselves to do more without realizing the toll it takes on them. To help me balance how I push myself on a given day, I wear a sleep tracker to gauge how well I sleep. When my sleep score isn't great, I'll scale back my workouts and take things a little easier. I don't want to put extra strain on my body.

While we may not all need the same amount of sleep, we all need to hit a certain number of sleep cycles to recover from the previous day's stress. In my experience, that number is 30 to 35 sleep cycles per week, each at a ninety-minute interval.

If you're really dialed in and practice sleep hygiene regularly, then chances are your sleep will generally be very good, even if you're only getting seven hours of sleep instead of eight or nine.

Types and Stages of Sleep

There are three types of sleep: light sleep, REM sleep, and deep sleep. We don't spend the bulk of our nights in deep sleep; in fact, we spend it moving through each of those three types.

Deep sleep is where the magic happens. It's the stage where recovery and repair take place. Approximately 25-30 percent of total sleep or around 1.5-2 hours of deep sleep per night often indicates a well-rested day ahead.

Sometimes we will be short on deep sleep if we're too restless, eat too late, or go to bed too late.

Sleep Hygiene

What wakes us up? More specifically, what makes us restless?

Often, it's light, noise, or a change in temperature. This is why we talk about dark rooms and trying to get phones out of the bedroom. Perhaps you've heard of or seen people blocking the lights on thermostats to soften the light impact, or using blackout blinds. All are efforts to reduce light interruption.

Personally, I find that temperature is huge for me. Women in menopause or perimenopause will also find temperature important. If they're too hot, they won't be able to get back to sleep.

The goal is to keep the room as dark and cool as possible.

For a lot of people, being too hot is one of the top things that will wake them up. Think about it. When have you heard someone say, "Oh, I couldn't sleep because it was too cold"? Even if the room is chillier than you'd prefer, you can always put a blanket on. I have my room set to around 18 degrees celcius, which does feel pretty cold, but it makes a big difference.

For sound, I often recommend a white-noise maker. Especially for women—whose brains are conditioned to pick up noises in the night, like that of a crying infant—it can be a major game-changer to have something that blocks out those smaller noises.

If you can control those three things (light, sound, and temperature), you can create an environment that better supports your sleep.

As I touched on already, our bodies produce melatonin in response to sunlight, aligning us with the sun's cycle. Morning exposure to sunlight—or red light—not only wakes us but triggers melatonin production for the evening.

You don't need a fancy lamp; simply going outside for 15-20 minutes after sunrise can help. Morning light exposure supports evening melatonin production and improves sleep. It's surprisingly effective.

Routines are also helpful. In my house, a couple of mornings per week I have to be at the clinic early, and some mornings I'm in charge of my kids. When I'm managing the kids, I get a chance to walk the dog after the sun rises.

Of course, every parent knows that not every day will go smoothly. On days when our morning routine falls apart, I use my red light and that helps me feel very alert.

Sleep Chronotypes

Have you ever thought you must not be sleeping right because you're not a morning person? You don't have to be a morning person to sleep well or be healthy, but you do need to live within your body's natural rhythm. When it comes to your natural sleeping rhythm, we call this your sleep chronotype.

Everyone is driven to sleep at different times of the day. Dr. Michael Breus, "The Sleep Doctor," identified four sleep chronotypes or natural sleep patterns. Some people are morning types, while others are not. Dr. Breus offers an online quiz to help you find your chronotype, allowing you to align your day with your natural rhythms. You can take it at: https://sleepdoctor.com/sleep-quizzes/chronotype-quiz/.

Your sleep patterns can guide how you spend your energy most effectively. For example, my chronotype suggests that my best workout energy isn't in the morning, so I avoid intense morning workouts. I'll do a little in the mornings, but I won't do a hard workout first thing. In fact, learning my sleep chronotype doesn't make me a morning person was a huge relief. For others, however, that first hour of wakefulness is their golden time for working out.

Robin Sharma wrote a very inspiring book about being a member of the 5:00 a.m. club. You'd wake up early, meditate, exercise, and intentionally start your day. It sounded ambitious and healthy, yet when I tried it, I felt awful.

Doing that routine just felt like it was going against my natural rhythms. When I found Dr. Breus's work, it confirmed what I'd always felt to be true: some of us are morning people, some are not, and not being one doesn't mean you're less healthy than someone who is.

Sleep isn't a one-size-fits-all metric. Not everyone will have energy in the morning, and not everyone who stays up past 10 p.m. is damaging their health (as long as they get enough sleep).

Knowing when you have more energy can also be helpful in your sleep practice. I know if I do a workout late at night or even yoga, it will energize me. I'll feel refreshed and ready to keep going, which isn't the best to help me calm down and get to sleep.

I have also noticed that my best workouts are a little later in the day versus first thing in the morning, so I tailor my resistance training schedule to the times best suited for me.

Biggest Obstacle

It's fascinating to me how many people will tell me they don't sleep well. They just say it like it's a thing they've learned to deal with, similar to what some of my patients will say about their pain. They just accept it, yet it affects how well they can get through the basics of life.

Dr. Matthew Walker, a professor at UC Berkeley's Center for Sleep Science, says the biggest obstacle he encounters when studying sleep is explaining its importance. And it is important. Shift workers who have constantly disrupted sleep schedules are more prone to health issues like obesity, diabetes, and heart disease. If you deprive mammals of sleep, you shorten their lifespan. That's significant!

Whenever someone comes into my practice and they're doing a good job with nutrition and exercise, the next question I ask is how they're sleeping. They could make small, easy, game-changing tweaks to their sleep hygiene, like adding magnesium supplements to their before-bed routine or starting a meditation practice to re-engage their parasympathetic nervous system.

The Vagus Nerve

One way we can access the parasympathetic nervous system is through the vagus nerve. If we stimulate the vagus nerve, we can induce a state of relaxation in the body.

The Latin root of the word vagus means "to wander," and that's just what this nerve does: It starts in the brainstem and travels through the body, wandering from your heart to your digestive organs and colon. It's constantly sending and receiving signals to help your body know when to switch to its rest-and-digest phase.

Again, if we needed to escape from danger, we'd want to be in the sympathetic nervous system, which will increase our heart rate and blood pressure, diverting blood away from our internal organs and toward our extremities so we can run faster.

However, within about an hour, you should get out of that response and back to a calm baseline.

When we're constantly triggered by stress responses all day long, however, our body stays in the sympathetic response. We need to help our bodies regain balance between these two systems.

Multiple ways exist for us to do that, each involving the vagus nerve.

Cold water to the face is a simple example. If you fill a sink with icy cold water and then put your face in it for fifteen to thirty seconds, that stimulates the vagus nerve. This might sound surprising since cold water feels like it should wake you up, but try it! I personally recommend taking a long, warm bath with Epsom salts followed by a cold shower (expose your face and neck to the cold water for 20-30 seconds).

Many home devices can help stimulate the vagus nerve. One I have used is a necklace with a small pendant that rests on your sternum called Sensate. When paired with specific music from the app, the Sensate will pulse with the bass, vibrating your sternum to stimulate the nerve. In this way, you can control the rate of the pulses with the song you choose.

As a chiropractor, I have a variety of techniques and hands-on approaches I use to stimulate the vagus nerve and create a relaxation effect in the body. The range of strategies available is vast, which means there's a method suitable for everyone's preferences and needs. These include:

1. **Vagus Nerve Reset**

   Lie on your back with your hands behind your head. Move your eyes only—keep your head still. Look to the right and hold for 30–60 seconds; then look to the left for the same duration. Visualize yourself stargazing to help focus.

2. **Relaxing Evening Activities**

   Avoid high-intensity exercises before bed. Instead, try calming rituals like applying lavender oil, drinking non-caffeinated teas like chamomile, or practicing meditation. These encourage relaxation and prepare your body for rest.

3. **Sing or Hum**

   Singing or humming stimulates the vocal cords and vagus nerve. Pair this with slow, deep belly breathing for maximum benefit.

4. **Box Breathing**

   Visualize a box as you breathe:

   – Inhale for 4 seconds

- Hold for 4 seconds
- Exhale for 4 seconds
- Hold for 4 seconds

Repeat, aiming to slow your breathing and reduce stress hormones.

5. **Extend Your Exhales**

   Focus on making your exhale longer than your inhale. This engages the diaphragm, promoting belly breathing and activating the parasympathetic nervous system. Chest breathing, by contrast, is linked to stress and trauma responses and engages muscles we want to relax. Another common breathing pattern is 4-7-8. Inhale for 4 seconds, hold that breath for seven seconds, and exhale slowly for 8 seconds.

6. **Facial and Jaw Massage**

   Gently massage your jaw and neck using small circular motions. This soothes tension and promotes relaxation.

7. **Tapping or Acupressure**

   Use tapping or apply pressure to key acupressure points to further calm your nervous system.

Sleep Scores

A variety of wearable devices are available that help track the quality of your sleep. For example, I use an Oura Ring, which provides me with a score for how my sleep for that night went.

Think about trackers in terms of a detailed sleep hygiene score; I wouldn't say the Oura Ring has transformed sleep for people, but it does give me an idea of my quantity, quality, and cycles of sleep. In fact, it factors total sleep, efficiency, restfulness, REM sleep, deep sleep, latency, and timing into my score:

- Total sleep refers to how much sleep one gets.
- Efficiency refers to the amount of time you spend asleep versus the time you spend awake. For example, if you take a long time to get to sleep or you wake up in the middle of the night and then can't get back to sleep, it will yield a lower sleep efficiency score.
- Restfulness is measured by movement. In essence, restfulness measures how much you moved or didn't move. Did you have to get up to go to the bathroom, for example? How much are you tossing and turning? All of that will be reflected in the restfulness component. Some trackers may not track restfulness, so if you're in the market for one, be sure to check.
- REM sleep is the phase in which we dream. If you get a lot of REM sleep, it helps reenergize your mind and body. As a benchmark, an optimal amount of REM sleep is about an hour and a half, but it decreases with age.
- Deep sleep is more restorative. It's where you rejuvenate and repair muscle damage from the previous day. Similar to REM sleep, the goal is to average about an

hour to an hour and a half. This is the state of sleep where everything drops: your blood pressure, breathing rate, and heart rate. It's really hard to wake up when you're in this stage of sleep, and if you do get woken up from it, you tend to be super-groggy. Deep sleep also happens earlier at night, which is why having a consistent sleep schedule is so important.

- Latency measures how quickly we fall asleep. It's obviously not good if it takes too long—no one likes lying in bed for ages. On the other hand, if you fall asleep two minutes after your head hits the pillow, it's a good sign you're overtired. (I do this sometimes, and it drives my wife nuts. She'll be there tossing and turning, and I'll be out cold.)

- Lastly, timing is all about the circadian rhythm and your sleep chronotype. In a nutshell, it monitors your bed time to see if it lines up with your sleep chronotype.

How you use the score is up to you. Personally, I pay attention to my sleep score to experiment and see what makes a meaningful improvement in my sleep or anything that has a negative effect.

For example, I will test different supplements and see if anything changes. It has also helped me to understand what affects my sleep negatively like late workouts, late meals, or alcohol.

Do I think everyone needs a sleep tracker to get their best sleep? No, absolutely not. If you have the money to spare, however, and you're curious about improving your sleep (and nerding out about its intricacies), I think it's a fun investment to make.

Creating a Good Sleep Environment

We all know that a dark room and a consistent wake-up time are the foundations for a good night's sleep. Room temperature is also important; I recommend sixty-six to sixty-eight degrees Fahrenheit (eighteen to twenty Celsius), though people also have success with cooler temperatures.

Avoiding caffeine after noon also helps set you up for sleep success later in the day. Some people will have a coffee at three in the afternoon, but that's really pushing it. The half-life of caffeine is six hours.

Let's say you have 100 mg of caffeine in your 3:00 p.m. coffee. At 9:00 p.m., you're still running on 50 mg of caffeine. That's still a significant amount of caffeine! It's enough to start affecting your sleep quality. That's why I set noon as a cutoff time.

Alcohol consumption is another area I'd limit before bed. My shift nurse patient, Stephanie, would often have a glass of wine or two late at night. While this would help her get to sleep, if she woke up in the middle of the night, she'd find it would be hard to get back to sleep.

With alcohol, specifically, it might relax you enough to fall asleep, but your liver still has to metabolize it. That, in turn, increases your heart rate, which gets you out of deep sleep, where the heart rate is slowed. I've noticed that if I have more than one glass of wine at night, my sleep scores tend to be bad.

These days, if I want to have a glass of wine, I try to have it with dinner so my body can process it better with food.

For Stephanie, we initially cut the wine out at night entirely. These days, if she decides to have a glass, she just makes sure she has it with dinner, and then it's a win-win: Stephanie still gets her wine, but now she gets a great night of sleep, too.

What We Add to the System

In this chapter, we've discussed addressing issues in our bodies from the inside. We have learned how the system operates and what influences it.

Next, let's examine what we bring into our bodies. What supplements are we taking? How do those affect and change our bodies? You don't have to be a biohacker and take seventy different supplements—that's a little too intense, even for me—but there are plenty of supplements that can improve the quality of our lives at low cost and with little inconvenience. They're easy to incorporate into our routines and don't cost a million dollars, a win-win situation for our bodies and budgets.

CHAPTER 8

Pillar Four: Supplementation

Chad was in his sixties and had markers of rheumatoid arthritis. As a result, Chad was so stiff he couldn't make a fist with one of his hands—that's how sore and inflamed his joints were.

Simple things we take for granted would be very difficult for Chad or cause him immense pain. Pulling up a zipper was a nightmare because he'd have to pull with one hand and then hold the bottom of the zipper closed with the other. Even putting on a shirt was a daily battle.

Chad was on multiple medications to try to lessen his pain, including one of the most powerful anti-inflammatory drugs out there.

When Chad came to see me, we went over his health history. "Are you on any supplements?" I asked.

"No," Chad said. "My doctor told me I don't need to take anything."

I decided to start small by encouraging him to try omega-3 fish oil. It's a relatively easy supplement to find and one most people tend to be, at the very least, a little deficient in. Chad rarely ate home-cooked meals, and when he did prepare food, it tended to be sandwiches and deli meats. He wasn't eating a high Omega-3 diet.

We worked together at the clinic, where I would adjust him and use other modalities available while he remained committed to taking a quality fish-oil supplement to enhance his diet. After a month, he could close that hand without wincing. That opened up so many everyday tasks for him! It was pretty amazing he could move his hand fully again, and to do so without pain was the icing on the cake.

After that, we both knew we should address his diet and nutrient intake more—after all, that was such a big win after a relatively small change! Chad fully bought in, and within another thirty days, he began to see some relief from the pain he'd lived with for years.

Sometimes, simple shifts can drastically change the course of your life. One sure did for Chad.

Basics of Supplements

If you recall from earlier in the book, we used to get most of our nutrients, vitamins, and minerals through our food. Now, things are different. Our farming practices have changed, and our soil, frankly, is exhausted. The high frequency of crop harvesting has contributed to fewer nutrients in the soil.

And it always comes back to the soil content.

Our agricultural processes have endured a massive shift. We use so many fertilizers and glyphosate—the active ingredient in RoundUp—in our foods that we can detect them in newborn babies. Again, these babies have not eaten anything: all their nutrition in life so far has come from what they received from their mothers.

Glyphosate, in particular, has been a hot-button topic because it's been linked to leaky gut syndrome. Interestingly, they don't use it in many countries in Europe. Some of my clients who can't eat bread and pasta in North America find they don't have any issues eating them when they travel to Europe; their bodies are simply irritated by the glyphosate present in North American grains. If they ingest it, they get bloated and cranky, their digestive system is a mess, their joints hurt, and everything aches.

The Environmental Working Group has lists of the "Dirty Dozen" and the "Clean Fifteen." The Dirty Dozen lists the most toxic fruits and vegetables based on their pesticide residue. Conversely, the Clean Fifteen are the top fifteen fruits and vegetables with the least pesticide residue. You can see the full lists at: https://www.ewg.org/foodnews/clean-fifteen.php.

The more we consume the standard North American diet of heavily processed foods, seed oils, and crops grown in depleted, chemically-laden soil, the unhealthier we become. Without supplementing what is lacking in our diet, it's almost impossible to become healthy in the long term. Returning to our backpack analogy, there's only so much weight our body can carry before it starts to sink.

Most of the food on the shelves in North America is out of control when it comes to additives, food chemicals, and other preservatives. It's engineered to last as long as it can and ends up having very little nutritional quality. Too many people assume that because they saw an ad for it on TV or it's on the shelf in nice packaging, it must be good for them. People read the side of a cereal box and see it's got all these vitamins added to it, which makes the cereal look good; what they're not asking is where those vitamins came from, how they were made, or what they're doing to our bodies.

With supplementation, our goal is to keep things simple. We look at what the body might be deficient in, and then, until we can get the bulk of the diet sorted out, we find ways to add what we're missing. Depending on geography, people in one place may be more deficient in certain nutrients than others.

For example, in Canada there is a higher percentage of people with MS than in Florida, Texas, and California. That's because Vitamin D deficiency increases the risk for MS. The farther north we live, the higher that likelihood.

Why do things like geography and soil content matter when talking about supplementation? Our macro and micronutrients come from what we consume, and what we consume can always be traced back to something that grows in soil. We'll talk more about macronutrients in the next chapter, but they are carbohydrates, fats, and proteins. Micronutrients are minerals and vitamins. We always want to be curious about where those come from, and what we may lack in our diets.

Starter Pack

So, where do we start with supplements? I don't want to recommend specific dosages because, depending again on where you live and what your body's needs are, they may differ from person to person. However, these are the top five supplements I feel most people could benefit from:

1. Vitamin D3

2. Omega-3s

3. Magnesium

4. Probiotics

5. Powdered greens

Note that with supplements, it's important to check the amount needed to see a benefit. For example, if you ask adults if they're taking a fish oil supplement, many will say yes. Many will only be taking one pill, however, when the supplement states you need to take three pills to benefit. Dosage is important.

So, before I dive into the different types of supplements, it may be helpful to know what to look for when checking amounts. On supplement packages, you'll see a number next to the acronym RDA. RDA stands for "recommended daily amount" and tells you the amount to take to avoid deficiency. While it's not individually optimized by any means, it can offer a good place to start for most people and then they can adjust their dose with their healthcare practitioner.

Vitamin D

Vitamin D is a general term to define fat-soluble vitamins that include both D2 and D3. It is an essential nutrient for optimal health that interacts with more than 3,000 genes. D2 comes from vegetable sources like mushrooms and is not as effective at raising blood levels as D3; therefore, D3 is the preferred form of supplementation. D3 is manufactured in the body when exposed to UVB rays and is found in some foods like fatty fish, fortified milk, and egg yolks.

Measuring blood levels is the most accurate way to determine your Vitamin D status. There are different units of measurement: ng/ml (USA) or nmol/L. It is generally accepted that levels below 30nmol/L or 20ng/ml are considered deficient and have serious health risks, including rickets. A blood level of 21-30 ng/ml or 50-75nmol/L is considered sufficient but can still create symptoms for some people.

Many experts in the Vitamin D field believe we should target the range of 40-60ng/ml or 100-150nmol/L to reduce preventable health issues. Research from Canada in 2009-2011 found the Canadian average to be 64nmol/L, which is considered sufficient for bone health but below the range for optimal health. In fact, suboptimal Vitamin D (less than 75nmol/L) is linked to bone and muscle issues, lowered immune function, poor mood and brain health, increased risk of chronic diseases like type 2 diabetes, high blood pressure, hormonal imbalances, and more. A 2010 study by Dr. William Grant concluded that if Canadians were to raise their Vitamin D levels to 105 nmol/L, it would save 14 billion dollars in healthcare spending and save 34,000 lives.

Even if you live in a place where you get a lot of sunshine and your Vitamin D is optimized for ten months of the year, it might be beneficial to find out which two months to consider supplementing.

What I find interesting is that culturally, we've been told to avoid the sun or wear sunscreen whenever we're outside. However, sunlight—specifically UVB rays—stimulates the body's natural production of Vitamin D, and sunscreen blocks this process.

The sun is the best source of Vitamin D we have, yet we have been told to avoid it. Obviously, we don't want to burn, but we need small amounts of sun exposure (10-30 minutes of midday sun, depending on where you live) to make Vitamin D naturally. For Canadians, the sun's rays are not powerful enough to manufacture Vitamin D naturally for approximately six months of the year.

One of the best things about Vitamin D is that it's impossible to overdose on it when you get it from the sun. If you make enough, your body simply stops manufacturing it to no ill effect. There's a group in the United States called Grassroots Health, which posts recommendations, articles, and research on Vitamin D. They also have home testing kits that I have used to track my levels.

Health Canada says the safe upper limit of Vitamin D3 supplementation is four thousand international units (4,000 IU's) a day, which makes it basically impossible to be toxic. Health Canada also says it is safe to supplement with this amount throughout the year.

Again, you can test with your doctor (or a company like Grassroots Health) to determine your levels and then figure out how much Vitamin D3 supplementation you need. Just by getting sufficient levels of Vitamin D3, you can significantly reduce your risk factor for MS and certain types of cancer. It was even a strong predictor of who might get hospitalized during the COVID-19 pandemic. I personally recommend testing your Vitamin D levels after the summer so you can experiment with supplementation in the fall and winter. We should try to target the ideal ranges mentioned above.

Various factors influence how much Vitamin D3 a person needs to supplement with, like gender and weight. Skin tone is also an important consideration; darker-skinned individuals produce less Vitamin D than people with lighter skin, so they should be especially careful when it comes to getting enough. Interestingly, I've also worked with some people from the Middle East—a place famous for its abundant sun—who have Vitamin D deficiencies because they spend so much time covered up in clothing.

Anyone taking Vitamin D3, however, should also take it with Vitamin K2 to help with absorption (many products contain them together). If taking separately, a typical dose of K2 would be 120mcg. You can also get K2 through fermented foods, egg yolks, and hard cheeses. Take your D3/K2 supplements in the morning or in the daytime.

Omega-3s

Omega-3s are another big deficiency. As we saw with Chad at the start of this chapter, adding an Omega-3 supplement like fish oil to your diet can move the needle for you within a quick time frame.

From an ancestral health perspective, the ratio between our Omega-6s and Omega-3s used to be two or four to one. Now, that ratio is twenty to one, possibly higher if you eat a lot of processed foods. The current ratio is literally ten times higher than what our bodies were designed to consume. Consequently, our bodies will be in a near-constant state of inflammation from all those oils—never mind all the sugars!

Part of how we make decisions about supplementing is understanding that we, as a society, have a baseline deficiency in certain vitamins and minerals. For example, unless you're eating cold-water fatty fish three to four times a week, as they do in Scandinavian countries, then you probably need to take an Omega-3 supplement.

Magnesium

Magnesium is commonly the number-one mineral deficiency for most people. We'll take a deeper dive into food in our next chapter, but because minerals come from what we eat and supplement with, it's helpful to go over it here.

It is recommended to get approximately 400mg/day to avoid deficiency. Also, it's considered a cofactor, meaning it participates in around 300 chemical reactions in your body, so having enough magnesium on hand allows your body to easily carry out those essential reactions.

The highest food sources from highest to lowest would include: pumpkin seeds, chia seeds, nuts like almonds and cashews, spinach, dark chocolate, avocados, black beans, salmon, and bananas. To attain approximately 400mg of magnesium, you could consume two tablespoons of pumpkin seeds, 1 ounce (a small handful) of almonds, 1 ounce of 85 percent dark chocolate, 1 medium avocado, and ½ cup of cooked spinach or black beans.

Unfortunately, when we consume a lot of grains in our diets, sometimes we struggle to absorb enough magnesium. Grains contain phytic acid, which can bind to minerals like magnesium so it can block their absorption, preventing our bodies from getting that mineral (this also occurs with zinc, iron, and calcium). It's strange to think that sometimes what we are eating (versus what we aren't eating) creates a deficiency, but magnesium is a case where that happens, especially when so much of the standard North American diet is grain-focused.

Caffeine is another thing that can inhibit magnesium absorption and can be another reason why someone might be deficient. Be sure to take your magnesium supplement about ninety minutes apart from coffee.

Some signs of magnesium deficiency are high blood pressure, headaches, and restless leg syndrome. What's tricky about magnesium is that because 99 percent of it exists in your bones, teeth, muscles, organs, and soft tissues, blood tests have a hard time picking it up, so it's difficult to measure a deficiency accurately.

There are also different forms of magnesium to consider. Two of the most commonly used forms are magnesium citrate and magnesium glycinate, both of which are safe for children and adults. Of the two, magnesium glycinate is the smaller molecule, so it tends to be easier for most people to absorb. A nice benefit of taking magnesium glycinate at night is it helps you sleep. Other forms that are well absorbed are malate and threonate.

The only side effect of magnesium supplementation (sometimes a beneficial one) is it gets the bowels moving. If someone has sluggish bowel movements and is interested in supplementing with magnesium, I'd especially recommend taking magnesium citrate.

Magnesium oxide is another variety that tends to be prescribed to people with constipation. It works by drawing water into the colon, but it has a low absorption rate, so it is less commonly used.

One common warning you'll see regarding magnesium is that sometimes we recommend people take it in divided doses, part in the morning and part at night, because too much at once may result in loose stool or GI upset.

And if you work out a lot, your body uses more magnesium. We need more magnesium to perform muscular activities, and we also lose electrolytes, including magnesium, when we sweat so be sure if you are performing a lot of exercise that you are sufficient in this essential mineral.

Magnesium also works synergistically with Vitamin D3 and K2 to increase the absorption of Vitamin D3 into your cells so they are often recommended to take together.

Check with your healthcare provider for dosing if you have a particular health condition or follow the instructions on your product label. Start slowly, focus on adding magnesium rich foods into your diet, and increase your added supplement dose to your GI and bowel tolerance.

Probiotics

The topic of probiotics is exciting because since the microbiome has gotten so much more attention in the last five years, people are making some really interesting discoveries in gut health. While people have understood for a long time that gut health is integral to overall health, we are only now understanding how that works.

Inflammation and poor mental health are also tied to gut health. The digestive system rules much more of the body than we have historically given it credit for. Part of why gut health is so fascinating is that the digestive tract is a single-cell layer. Its thinness makes it highly permeable—it's easy for nutrients to pass through, making it very sensitive to whatever we eat.

If the junctions between these two systems are tight (gap junctions, as we call them), then all is well. When the gap junctions become permeable, we start to have problems. Your body may recognize material leaking from the digestive system into the circulatory system as foreign bodies and initiate an auto-immune response to get rid of it.

Because this can be a huge issue, many people now test their gut health more frequently. Companies such as Viome

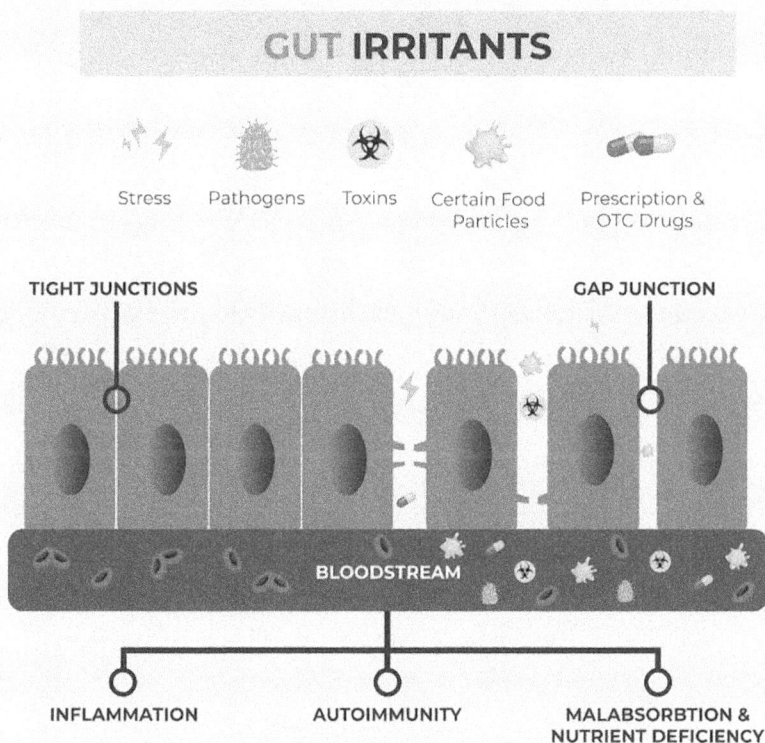

allow you to gain insight into what's going on in your gut. Considering that we're increasingly finding gut health linked to metabolic issues, the vast, sensitive system of the microbiome is rightly capturing the health community's attention.

Contrast this highly sensitive system with the typical North American diet full of sugars and grains. Sugar, specifically, can help promote the growth of unhealthy bacteria in the gut, as well as yeast. Because the gut microbiome is so carefully balanced, even small changes can have a big effect on the body.

For example, we now know that chronic fatigue is linked to gut health, as are Crohn's disease and IBS.

That said, taking a probiotic doesn't make everything in our digestive systems perfect automatically. Many different strains of probiotics are out there, and you may find that certain strains work better for your body than others. Some probiotics need refrigeration, others don't, and others are multistrain varieties. The options out there feel endless, which makes sense if you think about it. A person's microbiome is akin to their fingerprint: Each of us has a unique collection of gut flora that may respond differently to different foods. Check with your healthcare practitioner or talk to someone in your local health food store for options.

Many, many factors influence our microbiome on a daily level, and even the circumstances of our birth can change how it functions. When a baby comes through the birth canal in a normal vaginal birth, the baby gets its first exposure to healthy bacteria outside of its mother. Babies born through C-section don't receive this benefit, and they notably have higher rates of asthma. C-section births have also been linked to poor immune function and microbiome development.

As you can see, our immune system and gut health are very closely related. About 70 percent of our immune cells line our digestive tract, so the foods we eat matter a lot.

What can we do, then, to help our gut? An easy answer is to get more probiotics from fermented foods, specifically those without added sugars. Sugar, again, tends to skew gut health toward the negative, which is what we don't want to promote.

Good things to look for include kimchi, water or coconut kefir, kombucha, and plain yogurt.

The next thing to look for is the number of cultures. The cultures found in servings of yogurt tend to number in the millions, while those in a tiny probiotic supplement tend to be in the ten to fifteen billion range.

A good ballpark to look for in selecting a probiotic supplement is something in the ten to fifty billion culture range. The higher the number of cultures, the more likely they are to reach the colon.

If these numbers sound overwhelmingly large, consider what happens in your body when you go on antibiotics. As beneficial as it may be to solving a health crisis, one round of antibiotics will wipe out massive amounts of gut bacteria. Functional medicine doctors and naturopaths recommend ingesting fifty billion cultures per day over two weeks to recolonize the microbiome after something like that. That's just for one round of antibiotics.

Kids who have weaker immune systems from the start—maybe due to their C-section births—may be more prone to things like ear infections, for example, which sometimes require multiple rounds of antibiotics. When you think about what's going on with those kids' gut health, that can be really scary.

I do want to be clear: I am not saying to never take antibiotics, especially when the health situation is serious. Sometimes they are necessary and are the best course of action. Knowing the extreme effect antibiotics have on our gut health, however, it also makes sense not to request them for every cold or small inconvenience.

We already know that antibiotics won't help with viral infections. Worse, taking many courses of antibiotics without proper recovery time for the gut microbiome to repopulate between them results in lower immune function. People with repeated infections who return to antibiotics multiple times deplete their natural immune response.

If we want to have rockstar immune function, we need great gut health. Diet is a key piece of this, but probiotics can lend even more of a helping hand.

In addition to probiotics, we need prebiotics—what microbes need to feed. The prebiotics feed the "good guys" and help them flourish in the colon. Some probiotics have added prebiotics so you get both in the same capsule. While there's been some debate about whether probiotics can survive stomach acidity, some companies have added an enteric coating or time-delayed technology to assist in this process. Also, strains like lactobacillus and bifidobacterium are naturally acid resistant. Other strains like bacillus are spore forming, which helps them bypass the stomach acid and deliver into the colon. Take your probiotics with food to help assist in the delivery process.

Finally, with probiotics, it's important to get the right strains, vary your probiotic choices (to expose your gut to a variety of strains and cultures), and provide a good environment for them to populate the digestive tract. A good environment will depend on your nutrition. Again, a low-sugar environment is ideal.

Unhealthy bacteria will always exist in our digestive tracts; that is just a fact of life. However, when you have enough healthy bacteria, your body keeps the unhealthy bacteria in check.

It's a delicate, amazing system, and we owe it to ourselves to take care of it and keep it in the right balance.

Powdered Greens

The last item in our five-supplement starter pack is powdered greens. I recommend these because so many people struggle to meet the six to ten servings of fruits and vegetables a day that is recommended as part of a healthy diet. For busy people on the go, powdered greens offer a quick way to up their intake of nutrients and provide many benefits, including antioxidants. One scoop usually contains around the equivalent of six to ten servings of fruits and vegetables, so it's very easy to boost your overall health that way.

For kids and other picky eaters, powdered greens can be a godsend. If you eat very clean and don't have any issues getting in your recommended servings of fruits and vegetables, then you may be getting in all the micronutrients you need already without powdered greens. However, if you're not or have family members who struggle to, powdered greens provide a convenient, low-fuss way to get a lot of nutritional bang for your buck. You can put them in smoothies; they're often flavored and even come in single-size servings for convenience.

Most grocery and health food stores now have a whole section of them.

Another great thing about taking powdered greens is it reinforces the idea of adding things to your diet rather than subtracting them. It's easy to add powdered greens to a smoothie if you're already making one. Then you'll know your smoothie is helping your body by adding an extra boost of nutrition, which is just the cherry on top.

I often tell people health is a system of "pay now or pay later," meaning we can spend the extra money now on small to moderate ways to improve our health or pay for massive hospital bills and endure major illnesses later.

Ultimately, we can't put a value on anyone's health. These small changes add up in one way or another. Supplementing our diets with the Big Five—Vitamin D, Omega-3s, magnesium, probiotics, and powdered greens—costs about five dollars per person per day. It's a moderate investment that could have long-lasting benefits, especially later in life.

If you'd prefer to ease into supplementation, our starter pack list is also ordered in terms of priority. Vitamin D3 is such a big mover of health that it's worth addressing immediately (make sure to take with K2 as well). Fish oil and Omega-3s also have large effects on overall health. While magnesium is often the top mineral deficiency for most people, I list it third in my priorities because the benefits we derive from Vitamin D and Omega-3s can have a massive influence over our inflammatory levels, and thus, on preventing lifestyle diseases (also because it is possible to get adequate magnesium from the diet if you pay close attention to the magnesium rich foods listed above). If you eat very clean with little sugar, and have a variety of naturally occurring fermented foods, then you may not find you need to supplement with probiotics. A greens supplement may not be necessary for everyone—I offer them as suggestions for people who either have kids or who struggle to get a wide variety of greens into their diets.

Multivitamins

I have conflicted feelings about multivitamins. On one hand, it's very convenient to get all those nutrients in one place. On the other hand, it's tempting to sacrifice quality for convenience and take a multivitamin, like drugstore brands, with a coating your body can't break down and ingredients your body can't absorb. A good specific example of this is calcium. When calcium is in a low-quality multivitamin, it often comes in the form of calcium carbonate, which is basically limestone. Your body's ability to break that down and absorb it is very low!

Multivitamins often give us false confidence about how much we're helping our bodies. What's important to take away from this is that the form and delivery method of these micronutrients matter. We need to give our body things it actually understands how to process. Low-quality multivitamins often contain vitamins that won't be in the form your body can best use, and they have an inefficient delivery system because manufacturers try to make them as cheaply as possible.

Another problem is taking a lot of one vitamin or mineral without properly balancing it. For example, too much calcium and not enough magnesium can cause your arteries to harden. If calcium is correctly blended with magnesium, then both can be absorbed into the body better.

The body exists in a state of delicate balance, and that balance varies for everyone. It's tremendously hard for a one-size-fits-all multivitamin to check all the right boxes for every person who takes it.

Quality multivitamins are out there, but you have to do your research to find them. I typically take and recommend professional product lines that may be a bit more expensive, but those companies have invested the time and research into the correct forms of the vitamins and minerals. You get what you pay for!

My goal is to set you up so that even if you're not eating perfectly every day, you still have some protection from metabolic syndrome and the Big Four. A multivitamin, while a good idea in theory, will not be as effective as individually addressing the five suggestions we gave as our starter pack. It's much easier to balance individual supplements, and often, the quality will be much better when they're bought separately. The chance of finding a multivitamin that is balanced to you and has quality ways of delivering the micronutrients to your system is very small. If you aren't taking anything yet, start with adding a few things and then speak to someone knowledgeable in this area like a Naturopathic or Functional Medicine Doctor.

While that means keeping track of more capsules, you don't necessarily have to take every single supplement every day. Vitamin D3 and the Omega-3s in fish oil are fat-soluble, meaning your body can store them for a certain period of time. You could take fish oil three days a week, and you'd be fine. If you have trouble remembering to take things, you'll likely only need to take Vitamin D3 a few times per week and adjust the dose accordingly. For something more delicate, like the microbiome, you might want to take something daily just to keep everything in check. Water soluble vitamins, like Vitamin B, are processed quicker and don't remain in the body, so there's a limit to how much your body can actually absorb at a time. The same is true for magnesium; there's only so much magnesium you can absorb at a time before it begins to affect your GI system and bowels.

As I said before, it's a delicate balance. It may be more helpful to think of it as a ritual you're creating for yourself. Get in the habit of taking certain things at certain times. For example, you want to take your D3/K2 supplement in the day with some magnesium, omega-3, and probiotics with food, and any extra magnesium at night to assist with sleep. Some of my patients will take their greens product first thing in the morning while others will take it in the afternoon for a little energy boost. See what works for you and stay consistent!

Special Considerations

While the focus of this chapter has been on larger-scale issues, you may want to consider certain supplements based on your health history or the medications you're taking. For example, someone treating their acid reflux with a proton pump inhibitor (PPI) may find their levels of Vitamin B are lower than they should be as a consequence of their medication. That's okay; it's something we can easily address through evaluation and supplementation.

Even certain cholesterol medications, like statins, can create deficiencies in the body like Co-enzyme Q10 and Vitamin D3. Again, there may be a few extra things like CoQ10 that someone taking a statin might want to take. Check with your healthcare practitioner to ensure you can address your individual needs.

This chapter is not meant to be an exhaustive or comprehensive discussion on everything to do with supplementation, but rather a strong starting point for the curious beginner.

I cannot overstate the usefulness of having your levels of certain nutrients checked before you start supplementation. One company I have used to check my Vitamin D3 and omega-3 levels is Grassroots Health, but it's always a good idea to also check with your healthcare provider.

Small Changes Add Up

By choosing appropriate supplements for Chad, we restored the range of motion and mobility in both his hands. Where before he had very labored finger movements, he was eventually able to pull up his zipper and open jars with ease, and brushing his teeth was no longer a dreaded and monumental task. We turned things around for him in a matter of months.

That being said, patience is still a key factor. It's tempting to hope for results within the first week, but it takes time for the body to reset from prolonged inflammation. With enough consistency and time, the results can be pretty miraculous.

We're trying to set ourselves up with a certain level of protection from chronic disease so our longer time on earth also has a high quality of life. The easiest way to ensure that is through what we put into our bodies. While supplements are important to this, the bulk of how we nourish ourselves is through our food. The cleaner we can get our diets, the less we'll need to rely on outside sources to provide what our bodies need for optimal health. After all, why spend all this time on fixing deficiencies when we can simply prevent them from happening in the first place with our diet?

CHAPTER 9

Pillar Five: Food

Gordon was in his seventies and one of those guys who always had a pretty obvious belly. His health wasn't in the best place (he was a Type 2 diabetic), so he'd signed up for one of my six-week, in-person workshops where we try to reduce sugar intake. If you've visited my website, you may have seen the Five-Day No Sugar Challenge, which pretty much does what it says: You commit to not eating foods with added sugars for five days and see how it makes you feel.

The in-person program is similar, except it lasts six weeks and allows participants more time to ease off sugar—and Gordon was all in.

He worked hard over the six-week period of the course, found that he was losing weight, and decided he wanted to continue on with a reduced sugar intake. Losing a little bit each week, he lost fifty pounds after 6-8 months just by consistently eating healthily! In the months after he started the program and continued to eat well, he was also able to get off his insulin. This was a major win for him; before the substantial weight loss, he had all the markers of a heart attack waiting to happen. Gordon kept feeling better and better, so he stuck with it. His arthritis symptoms even went down, and all seemed well.

Then the pandemic happened.

Gordon came back to the clinic a few months after it was safe to do so, seeking neck pain relief. Over the course of the next few months, I started to notice him putting on weight— not a lot, but a little bit each visit. Eventually, I brought it up and asked if we could weigh him.

While he was still thirty pounds below his heaviest, he'd gained back twenty of the pounds he'd lost in our program. He knew his blood sugar wasn't in a good place, either. I asked him if he understood what was happening inside his body when his blood sugar was off. He did.

He'd just lost his motivation, like so many of us did during COVID-19.

So, I had to give him the "scary talk." Did he want a heart attack? Because that was what was coming if he persisted with his current path.

Gordon was someone I'd thought had it figured out. He'd worked hard, lost the weight, and it seemed like he was keeping it off. Then he got lax. The day we had our hard conversation, his wife even thanked me for bringing it up with him. While Gordon wasn't sneaking food, he had started eating more things he shouldn't. Because he's naturally insulin resistant, those processed foods are essentially poison to him. They're only going to put him more at-risk for bad things happening later on. Gordon knew all this, but he needed a reminder to get back on the right track.

The Most Heated Debate in Health

Food habits are always the hardest for people to change. Period.

If you go into a bookstore right now, you'll find an array of diet books promoting eating styles that promise they're the most effective way to lose weight: vegan, carnivore, vegetarian, keto——each one promises theirs is the way to go. So, what's the answer?

I'm not going to use this chapter to present you with a strict black-and-white list of what to eat and what not to eat. What I want is to give you a framework of general principles you can work off of and adjust to your own body.

My goal is to help you cut down on or eliminate the big issues, those processed and fast foods, and then leave it to you to tailor your own perfect diet.

When it comes to what's right, professionals in the field— including PhDs, MDs, and researchers—all seem to take different sides. People like Joe Rogan and other podcast celebrities hotly debate whether or not a vegan athlete can be competitive. For the average person, all this argument and scholarly disagreement is too much to sift through. That's why I got additional certifications as a health coach and nutrition coach— so I could deepen my understanding of nutrition and the best way to teach my patients.

As a healthcare professional, I have tried to watch and read everything I can on the subject of health. I want to understand where all these people are coming from and what makes their diet choices work so well for them. For example, if someone promotes a vegan diet as what keeps them healthy, I want to know what specifically about it delivers on that promise. There's a lot of research that says eating vegan can help reduce heart disease, but that's also when it's being compared to the standard North American diet. Unfortunately, the standard North American diet is so bad that almost any change will be healthier for you.

What I have found from twenty-plus years in practice and helping thousands of patients is that different diets work for different people. There may not be a single diet that is one-size-fits-all right for everyone. Different bodies like different things. While you may be able to, through careful experimentation, find the perfect diet for yourself, chances are that diet won't be perfect for someone else. This is especially true with food sensitivities and allergies.

For example, it would be easy to recommend the Mediterranean diet because there's a ton of research on its effectiveness. However, if a person is sensitive to tomatoes, eggplant, and other nightshade vegetables, then it won't be a good match for them. Eating those kinds of foods consistently may create inflammation in their body.

Another good example is kale. Many people recommend eating kale, but what they don't know is that kale is high in oxalates. If you're a person who isn't sensitive to those, then you can eat all the kale you want. If you are sensitive to oxalates, it may lead to kidney stones.

What's a person to do?

There's always going to be something that doesn't work for you that works for someone else and vice-versa. For my own body, I've found that occasionally following a ketogenic diet has been really beneficial. I have insulin resistance in my family, so being able to ease off carbohydrates for three to six weeks at a time is very helpful to me in maintaining my health. Most of the time I will follow what I recommend here later in the book. I've also done vegan cleanses once or twice a year and had good results (though I've also watched people follow a vegan diet and seen their health deteriorate due to unhealthy choices—French fries are vegan, after all).

Again, a lot depends on what your particular body's needs are. Much of how we learn these things is by experimenting. What does your body feel best eating? What doesn't make it feel good? You also have to consider what your genetic weak spots might be and eat the foods that will best support your health long-term.

Processed Foods

I would be remiss if I didn't talk about processed foods and their impact on our culture and collective diets.

First off, our general working definition of a processed food is a food that an outside company has assembled. Or, in other words, a food that has to be put together from multiple sources versus having a single origin.

For example, it's easy to see that beef comes from a cow and that an apple comes from a tree. Those are whole foods, and their origins are easy to trace. Applesauce in a jar may come from apples, but it may also have sugars and other chemicals added in. Beef ravioli in a can certainly has beef, but it likely also contains preservatives, sugars, and an assortment of added industrial seed oils to help it taste better and extend shelf life.

So, what's wrong with all those chemicals, seed oils, and sugars? Our body doesn't process them very well. It takes a long time for the body to figure out how to break those foods down, what it can use, and what it needs to discard. Those chemicals and preservatives accumulate and end up hanging around in our bodies for a long time, causing inflammation.

Don't worry—there's an element of grace to this. We understand that processed foods aren't the best for us healthwise, but many of them are still very delicious. At the end of the day, we want to build a sustainable and enjoyable diet for ourselves. That may mean following the 80-20 Rule, where 80 percent of what we eat is clean, whole foods, and then we give ourselves 20 percent of space for other foods we enjoy. For some people, the 90-10 Rule is better. It all depends on what your body needs and what your long-term health goals are.

Some people may find it easier to cut out processed foods entirely for shorter spans of time. As I touched on in Chapter 4, for them, it's often much easier to do something at 100 percent compliance than at 95 percent because there's no need to ask questions or wonder. If you're cutting out processed foods entirely for six weeks, the decision has already been made for you.

No matter what you do, you have to be congruent: Your daily choices matter, and they have to be in line with your goals.

My issue with many diets is they are hard to maintain over the long haul. While they can serve as effective "reset buttons," they often fall short in terms of sustainability. For instance, you might successfully eliminate added sugars for a few weeks, only to find yourself craving them again. Some people can reintroduce sugars in small amounts, while others need to abstain completely because they're physically and emotionally addicted to sugar.

While calling it an addiction may seem over the top, it's really not. There's a cycle of craving, satisfying the craving, getting the reward neurochemicals, and then feeling better. That's incredibly difficult for people to break out of.

The advantage of cutting something out entirely is it eliminates decision fatigue, the exhaustion that comes from repeatedly making the same choices. My personal strategy involves setting short-term dietary goals, like committing to a specific eating pattern for a week or two. Once these decisions are made, there's no need to deliberate over every meal. This method can be crucial for individuals striving to achieve their health objectives.

It's a tough balance to strike. We don't always see what's going on inside our bodies, so it can be easy to take the warning signs less seriously.

And I get it: This is an intimidating process. But moving away from processed foods is the single most important shift you can make in your nutrition toward achieving better health overall.

What scares me most is people thinking they have the luxury of time. They feel okay, even if their habits may not be very healthy, and that's not enough impetus to change. Their doctors may warn them they're at higher risk for a heart attack, but because they don't feel unhealthy, they don't take action. For 60 percent of heart disease victims, the first sign of a problem is a heart attack.

That was the case for my dad. We had no clue, no idea that heart disease was a problem for him. It came out of nowhere and ended his life.

There *is* a degree of urgency to this. Your health isn't something that can be procrastinated upon or postponed until a more convenient time. The actions you take now, today, matter.

And hands down, optimizing your nutrition is one of the most powerful ways to increase your longevity.

Just *how* powerful is food?

For me, the first area I start to attack with a new client in their sixties or seventies isn't exercise; it's food. I know I can change their life more drastically if we focus on getting their food choices dialed in much more than trying to get them to start a running program or getting into the gym.

For example, most people who are at risk for Type 2 diabetes can get their blood sugar back within a healthy range within six to eight weeks of eating properly. I've seen it at my clinic. Food is literally the fastest way to get things back under control.

Food in the Modern World

Food in the last few hundred years has changed a lot. If you look at pictures of people sixty, even fifty years ago, few people were obese. The obesity epidemic really started in the seventies and the eighties when we started to promote whole grains to the base of the food pyramid. Suddenly, grain-based carbohydrates and processed foods became a staple in North American diets.

What you eat and how it affects your body is often influenced by both geography and genetics. Nutrition that works for someone in the tropics will likely not work for someone living in the Arctic. Someone from the Arctic, for example, probably has a higher saturated fat diet because of their environments, yet heart disease isn't an issue for them. Meanwhile, people from Africa may eat a diet rich in carbohydrates and fruit and still stay fit and thin.

Interestingly, if you take someone genetically designed to eat a higher fat content and place them in an environment where they eat more carbohydrates, they will very quickly develop metabolic issues, like Type 2 diabetes.

Despite this, our fundamental nutritional needs likely remain the same, centered around plant-based foods and proteins. However, sticking to such diets long-term can be challenging for many.

So, what's changed in the last hundred years? It's not our genes—it's our lifestyles. We now have access to a wider variety of foods than ever before, with processed foods being a relatively recent addition to our diets. One of the biggest challenges we face today is assuming that if something is readily available in stores or advertised on TV, it must be safe. While technological advancements have boosted food production and shelf life, the additives used may have negative long-term effects on our health.

This over-processing of grains, starches, and sugars has led to chronic illnesses like Type 2 diabetes and the obesity epidemic. Chronic preventable disease remains the largest challenge to our health as a whole. I don't think that will ever change. So that's why we start with reducing sugars and processed foods as our foundation.

The trick to health through food is to eat as naturally as we can.

What Exactly Is "Clean Eating"?

Before we dive into the topic of clean eating, I want to emphasize that you shouldn't view this as a detox or a cleanse, but rather a lifestyle shift toward eating healthier.

For something that sounds like it should be relatively easy to define, in practice, clean eating is a lot harder to pin down. So, to walk you through it, I'll cover what it is, what it isn't, how to do it, and what to watch out for.

To understand clean eating, it's helpful to define what it isn't. Again, clean eating isn't about strict deprivation or following fad diets. Clean eating is mindfully choosing whole and well-sourced foods and involves removing foods with added sugars, especially those found in processed and fast foods.

How to Do It

First, I want you to reconnect with your *why*. It's not easy to change the way you eat, so connect with your deeper reason and use that as the foundation for your next steps.

Start by focusing on fresh, whole foods found around the perimeter of grocery stores, such as produce, meat, dairy, and eggs. Additionally, adhering to lists like the Clean Fifteen and Dirty Dozen can guide your food choices. Try to prioritize organic options for items with higher pesticide residue.

"Clean" also extends into animal products. I always recommend you eat the cleanest source of animal protein you can afford. Why? Because, at the end of the day, you are consuming whatever the animal you're eating once ate. If you eat beef, for example, and the cow your beef came from was fed corn, soy, and high amounts of Omega-6, then the meat you eat will contain those spiked values of Omega-6. On the other hand, if you look at cattle fed on grass and natural pastures, their meat has much higher values of Omega-3, the good fatty acid, and normal amounts of Omega-6. A lot of the studies that link red meat to cancer don't often take into consideration where the protein is coming from. As we can see, it matters.

Likewise, the same metric applies to seafood. The key words you'll look for here are wild caught. If your salmon was farmed, it may have been fed a whole bunch of soy and antibiotics neither of which you want in your dinner. Part of clean eating is also paying attention to the food chain like that.

This may be more expensive than what you normally pay at the grocery store, but it's an investment in your health. The added chemicals you put into your system can stay in your system and become just another stressor for your body to deal with. That's what we're trying to prevent.

What to Watch For

When trying to eat clean, perhaps one of the most shocking things about grocery shopping is learning to read the labels on your food and realizing that sugar is *everywhere*.

Pick up a can of pasta sauce and look at the nutrition facts on the back. Whoa! How are there so many grams of sugar in there? It doesn't even taste sweet! It's the same with barbecue sauce, ketchup, and cereal. Even yogurt, which people tout as supposedly good for you, has fifteen to twenty grams of sugar.

The World Health Organization recommends no more than 20-40 grams (about 5-10 teaspoons) of free sugar—this is added sugar and sugars from honey, fruit juices, and syrups—per day for adults. For kids, that's even lower. To put this into context, one twelve-ounce can of Coke has 39 grams.

Not all sugars are equal. While the natural sugars in fruits are generally healthier than added sugars, they still contribute to overall sugar intake. However, the World Health Organization (WHO) distinguishes between naturally occurring sugars, like those in whole fruits, and free sugars, which include added sugars and those in fruit juices. Free sugars are what count toward the recommended intake limits.

How you consume sugars also matters. For example, eating an orange is not the same as drinking orange juice. Orange juice contains more concentrated sugars and lacks the fiber that slows sugar absorption in whole fruits. Additionally, it's easier to drink excess calories than to eat them. This is why it's so important to be mindful of sugary beverages (like that can of Coke!) and their impact on your overall sugar consumption.

A person with a lot of weight to lose should focus on cutting down on additional sugars. A more active person may find their tolerance for carbohydrates is slightly higher, given their body has to use them to sustain their higher energy levels.

And try not to get too caught up on being perfect all the time. Don't forget the 80/20 or 90/10 Rules. You may not be able to control what's available at parties or events, but remember that your environment affects your success, and you can control what you eat at home.

When trying to eat clean, reading labels gives you the power to make a more informed choice. Once you know how much added sugar is in processed food, it's easier to shift away from that.

So, when we look at labels, our first goal is to be aware of the sugars hidden in our foods. Our second goal is to find what's going to give us the most protein for our buck. Speaking of protein, let's take a closer look at why it's an important macronutrient.

Shifting What You Eat

Balanced nutrition involves understanding the three main macronutrients—proteins, carbohydrates, and fats—while focusing on whole, minimally processed foods. When we break down food into these general categories and then set goals for how much we want to eat of each, it gives us a lot of choice in which specific foods we pick to achieve that.

Protein

Eating enough protein is a hot topic right now in the health community, and rightly so. Today, most of the experts I follow and talk to are saying that eating 0.7 to 0.8 grams of protein per pound of body weight is the most ideal amount to maintain a healthy weight. If we're talking about weight loss, we'd actually want to be eating even more protein (close to 1g per pound of ideal body weight). I'll talk about why later. If our goal is to maintain good muscle mass, then we'd shoot for about one gram of protein per pound of body weight.

So, for a person who's 200 lbs., I'd recommend something like 140 grams of protein a day. Now, someone might get nervous and say that seems like a lot, especially given the correlation between high protein intake and kidney issues. A sustained, very high protein diet, such as 2-4 grams per pound, might cause kidney problems down the line, but 0.7 to 0.8 grams per pound of body weight will not. We're in a safe range here.

And as I touched on in the last section, be mindful of where your protein sources come from and try to eat the best quality protein you can afford.

Carbohydrates

Carbohydrates cover a wide range of foods. When we say carbohydrates, most people assume we're talking about grains and starches, like pasta, bread, and cereals. In reality, carbohydrates are energy producers for the body, and while they do appear in bread and pasta, we can also get them from fruit and vegetables.

And since there's no nutritional advantage to eating grains over fruits and vegetables, your goal should be to meet your carbohydrate needs first with vegetables, then fruits. Vegetables are a priority because they have a lower glycemic index, meaning they have less impact on blood sugar compared to some fruits. While fruits like berries are lower in glycemic index than some vegetables (like carrots) and also provide fiber, they contain fructose, which is processed differently by the body. Overeating fructose can strain the liver, which is not an issue with vegetables. Vegetables also provide extra fiber, making them an excellent choice for improving health after moving away from processed foods.

I also want to note that carbs in and of themselves aren't bad; but when you reduce them in your diet, you'll likely see your blood sugar go down and receive other significant health benefits.

When I speak with clients about carbs, bread is what they usually ask me about the most. "What if I make my own bread?" they ask.

Well, if you're in good shape and hitting all your health goals, then some bread every once in a while is fine. It's not going to kill you. If you make it from scratch and you're using organic flour, then you're not getting as many chemicals so you're probably okay on occasion.

Remember also that your carbohydrate intake should be tailored to how well your body processes carbohydrates and your activity level and age. For example, I never think about how much fruit my kids eat, but I do think about how much protein they get since they are starting to work out and growing all the time. But if someone has Type 2 diabetes and they are fairly inactive, they need to be more careful.

That being said, I like to keep things simple. I also think it gives people a unique window into how they might feel if they experimented and removed certain food groups, like breads, from their diets. Long-term, we're trying to choose foods that have the least effect on our blood sugar and to manage inflammation. Carbohydrates tend to be the main foods that affect both, so I recommend going with mostly vegetables and being selective about which fruits you choose to eat. Typically, berries are the safest choices, especially organic ones.

Healthy Fats

Our bodies use fats to absorb certain vitamins and build cell membranes, so we want to make sure we're fueling our systems with enough healthy fats to do that. Consuming the wrong kinds of fats can cause inflammation. Our goal is generally to try to increase our Omega-3 content, and our healthiest fats come from fish, especially fatty fish like salmon and sardines.

Other healthy fats—though not high in Omega-3s—are olive oil, avocados, coconut oil, and grass-fed butter. Those things make up 80-90 percent of the oils I regularly consume.

An added benefit to olive oil is it's really good for salad dressings and dips. Just make sure you choose one that is cold-pressed and stored in a dark bottle. If you put it in the fridge, it should harden. When it comes to cooking, don't cook olive oil on high heat. If it starts to smoke and smell bad, that's the oil going rancid. For higher temperature cooking or frying, I recommend using coconut oil, avocado oil, or butter.

We also touched on the importance of Omega-3 in the previous chapter—most people aren't eating fatty fish three times a week, so this is a prime place to supplement as well.

Plenty of options also exist for the vegetarians out there. Hemp, chia, flax seeds, and walnuts are all great sources of healthy fats without animal products.

Ultimately, fats end up being pretty simple. If the fat isn't coming from one of the sources I listed above, then it's something you should minimize.

But What About Fiber?

One of the major advertising strategies for cereals has been that they're high in fiber. We've seen so many links between different kinds of cancers and a high-processed food and low-fiber diet that it inspires us to get more fiber.

The good news about fiber is if you're getting most of your carbohydrates from vegetables, you're already hitting your fiber goals. That's part of the beauty of a vegetable-focused approach to carbohydrates: you don't have to worry about all the little details of "Am I getting enough fiber?" or "Am I getting all the micronutrients and minerals my body wants?" It's all right there in the food you're already eating.

Pretty convenient, right? When you give the body what it needs, it makes your life a lot easier.

What If I Can't Go Cold Turkey?

Quitting processed foods is a bold step, so it's understandable if it feels overwhelming. Many of us have grown accustomed to them over a lifetime. Maybe you're not one for abrupt changes, or perhaps you've just become aware of the hidden sugars in the typical North American diet. Don't panic or feel like you have to do it all at once—or worse, give up feeling like a failure. Nutrition is deeply ingrained, often tied to emotions or even belief systems.

Think about what works for you and where your current health is at. Are you the kind of person who needs small, incremental changes to ease into a bigger change? Do you have the time to gradually commit? Or are you a person who needs to make a big change? Do you get discouraged and quit when you don't see results and run out of momentum? Many find success in committing to significant changes for a set period, then reevaluating. Knowing it's not forever can be reassuring, allowing occasional treats without guilt.

Again, it matters less what you do 10 percent of the time. What matters is what you do in the remaining 90 percent. If 90 percent of your diet consists of clean vegetables, fruits, and protein with a focus on healthy fats, you're doing a great job.

The biggest battle I usually have to face with clients is getting past all those processed foods. What do you buy at the grocery store out of habit? When do you tend to stop for fast food? If you grab a coffee, do you automatically grab a muffin as well? This is a good chance to take an inventory and figure out what your eating habits tend to be.

It's always easy to say you eat pretty clean. When you go through the lists of what you actually are eating, however, does that assertion still stand up? If it doesn't, then you have your first step laid out for you.

Again, don't sweat it if you're feeling intimidated. Give yourself a time frame to work with, tell yourself this isn't going to be forever, and see how your body reacts.

You might be surprised by how good you feel.

Hydration

Water intake is another popular topic in wellness spaces. It has a place when talking about overall nutrition because it helps regulate body temperature, aids in digestion, flushes out toxins, and supports various bodily functions.

So, how much water should you be drinking?

An easy rule of thumb is to try to drink half your body weight in ounces each day. If you weigh 200 pounds, that's about 100 ounces or three liters. For most people, this number will fall between 2.5-3.0 liters of water per day. If you drink caffeine, the amount changes.

Caffeine is a diuretic. That means it dehydrates you. For any number of caffeinated beverages you have, you need to add that amount of water *extra* to your daily amount. It's a one-for-one exchange.

Electrolytes

Electrolytes are the minerals that help keep water in your body, like sodium, potassium, and magnesium. That retention is good because if you keep drinking water, eventually your body will reach a point where it's saturated and it'll just start peeing it out. With electrolytes, we can keep more of that water in our bodies and help ourselves stay hydrated. If we want to get more of that water into our cells, then electrolytes are the answer.

Sodium, in particular, is the dominant electrolyte. That might explain why we've become obsessed with sea salt as a society—it's not just because it tastes really good! It's actually doing good stuff for our bodies as well. Salt helps keep water inside our bodies. It also helps our blood volume maintain its water balance.

Consequently, to reap these benefits, you need a certain amount of sodium in your body. If you quit eating processed foods, you will need to add some sodium back into your diet.

It's all about balance. Too little or too much salt can have a deleterious effect.

What happens when your electrolytes are out of balance? As you start to decrease your carbohydrate intake, you might experience dizziness and lightheadedness if you're not getting enough salt. Ingesting fewer carbs will lower your insulin levels and that means you'll often excrete more water. You actually have to increase your salt and electrolyte intake or you'll just be peeing all the time, as well as dealing with being lightheaded and dizzy.

People also experience problems with exertion and lack of energy with low electrolytes on a lower carbohydrate diet. For example, they'll go for a run or try to work out and feel absolutely exhausted. Maybe they have more frequent headaches. Those are all signs you need more salt and electrolytes.

What I often see in these situations is that people reduce their sugar intake even more, sometimes blaming headaches on a sugar detox. While it's true that less glucose in the body leads to lower insulin levels, causing us to excrete more water, the real issue isn't just the lack of glucose. The problem is that we're not compensating for it by giving our bodies enough salt and electrolytes to maintain balance.

That's why I often recommend that people who are switching to a lower carbohydrate diet also have a quarter teaspoon of salt for every liter of water they drink. You barely even notice the taste if you put that amount in a big jug of water. Alternatively, you could also add two or three dill pickles and a handful of green olives.

With electrolyte drinks, we have to be a little more careful because many of the options available on the market have a ton of added sugars. You want to avoid as many artificial sweeteners and added chemicals as possible.

To recap: When it comes to overall hydration: 1) Make sure you're drinking enough water (and don't forget to account for caffeine), and 2) Add in a high-quality salt with a good micronutrient content if you're following a low-carb diet. (Examples would be Redmond or Baja Gold.)

If you'd like to check out some further reading on this subject, I recommend *The Salt Fix* by Dr. James DiNicolantonio. Dr. DiNicolantonio is a researcher and pharmacist, and his area of expertise is electrolytes and hydration, so I often refer to him. In essence, his thesis says don't blame salt for the problems that sugar created.

Artificial and Alternative Sweeteners

Is an artificial sweetener less harmful than regular sugar? I get asked this question a lot, especially when it comes to sodas. Are diet sodas really better than their regular counterparts? I hate answering questions like that. Many think they can consume as many diet sodas as they want because they don't contain as much sugar; that just isn't true. Sure, if you're a diabetic, then diet soda will be better, because it has fewer sugars. But neither is great for you!

While maple syrup is also natural, it's very high in sugars. Compared to refined sugar, yes, maple syrup is definitely the better choice; but it's similar to the regular soda versus diet scenario. Maple syrup isn't the best choice out there; it's just better than the standard North American diet's adherence to refined sugar.

For example, in a teaspoon of maple syrup, there's about five grams of sugar. If you had three teaspoons, then you'd have half your added sugar allowance for the day. That's a lot in a very small package!

I tend to avoid sweeteners like aspartame and the like. These are found in everything from "no sugar added" yogurt to different baking products, and even to protein powders. In truth, we don't know enough about them to determine whether their long-term effects on the body will be negligible.

Try These Instead

If you have to get your "sweet" on, I usually recommend sugar alcohols or stevia. Stevia is a plant that's four hundred times sweeter than sugar. Talk about a little going a long way! It usually comes in a powdered or droplet form, and is so sweet you literally cannot use it as a one-to-one replacement. Erythritol is another one that often comes in combinations that can be swapped out one-for-one with sugar, making it easy to use as a substitute in recipes. The taste is similar, too.

Sugar, maple syrup, and honey are easy to swap for stevia and erythritol. Personally, I have found that stevia and erythritol work well together. There's also a plant called monk fruit from Asia that's extremely sweet and is available in drops or powder, too.

It's somewhat controversial and debatable whether artificial sweeteners have negative long-term effects, but I think it's saying something that most of the doctors I follow in the natural health space tend to stay away from them.

I also want to be careful here not to polarize anyone away from certain foods or to demonize eating anything. So much depends on your activity level and physical health. Are bananas bad? On the whole, no. Is it okay for an active kid on his way to hockey practice to snack on one? Absolutely. Is it okay for a diabetic to have two or three of them a day? No because that could cause a large swing in blood sugar. We have to be prepared to work with our bodies, not against them.

Finding ways to satisfy your sweet tooth without spiking your blood sugar can be a big transition to make. Everyone is afraid to give up the sugar. I get it. Part of me running through all these artificial sweeteners is to give you alternatives so that moving away from sugar doesn't feel so scary or intimidating anymore. I'm not saying you can't have those indulgences you like, but remember to keep your food choices consistent with your goals.

Why We Care About Blood Sugar

We've talked a lot about the importance of not causing our blood sugar to rise too much. Now might be a good time to dig more into the science behind how that and insulin responses are related.

One reason I talk to my patients about trying not to consume too much sugar at one time is because your body can only deal with so much sugar in the bloodstream at once. Let's briefly look at how this works. When you consume sugar (sucrose), your body breaks it down into fructose and glucose (this is what circulates in your bloodstream). Glucose is used by your body for energy, and when it's available in large amounts, your body has to process it quickly.

THE GLYCEMIC INDEX

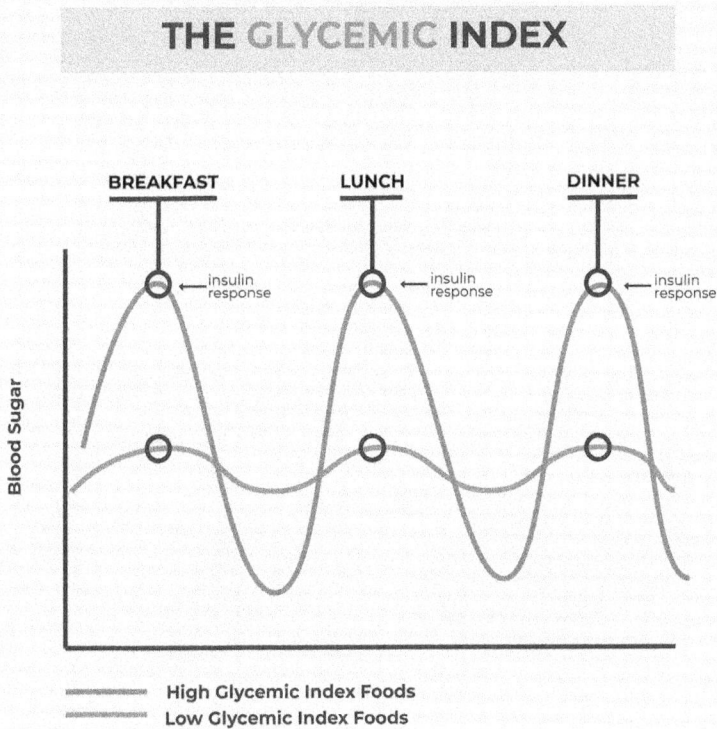

Over time, this high sugar intake can strain our system and raise our risk of developing Type 2 diabetes. If you have a family history or a genetic predisposition to insulin resistance—when your body loses the ability to efficiently shuttle glucose into cells—this overconsumption of sugar can further stress your body. As a result, glucose builds up in the bloodstream, leading to higher blood glucose levels and increased insulin production. Since insulin is a fat storage hormone, these strong insulin responses signal the body to store more fat and make it harder to lose the fat we already have.

Also, I want to emphasize how these problems with insulin resistance are connected to so many other health issues like the Big Four (cardiovascular disease, diabetes, cancer, and neurodegenerative diseases). Most people are not aware of the vast effects this insulin mechanism has on our overall health.

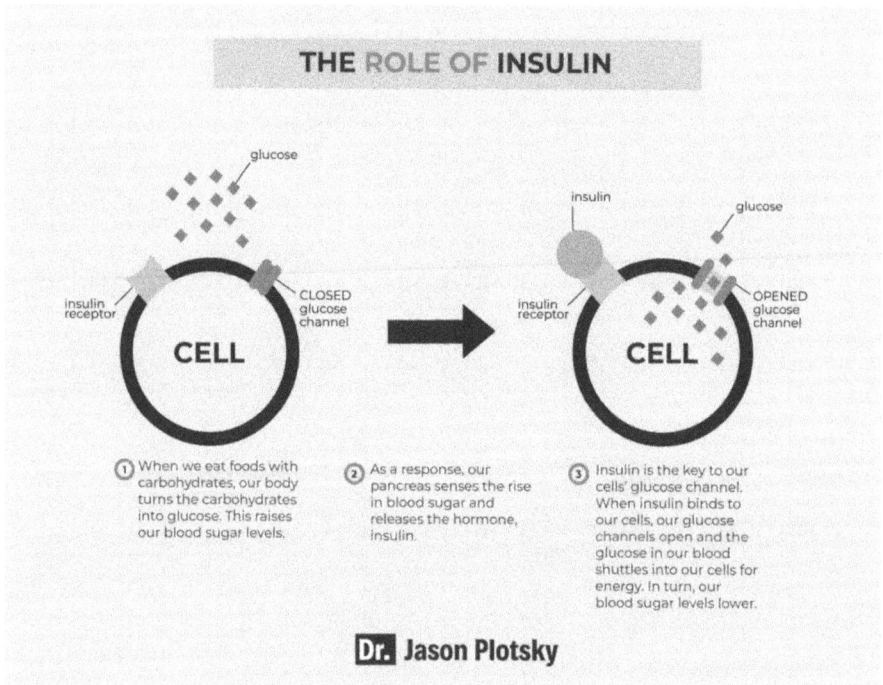

THE ROLE OF INSULIN

glucose

insulin

glucose

insulin receptor

CLOSED glucose channel

insulin receptor

OPENED glucose channel

CELL

CELL

1. When we eat foods with carbohydrates, our body turns the carbohydrates into glucose. This raises our blood sugar levels.

2. As a response, our pancreas senses the rise in blood sugar and releases the hormone, insulin.

3. Insulin is the key to our cells' glucose channel. When insulin binds to our cells, our glucose channels open and the glucose in our blood shuttles into our cells for energy. In turn, our blood sugar levels lower.

Dr. Jason Plotsky

To understand it a little better, let's talk about how our bodies store energy. If you've eaten in the last 1-2 hours, then there's glucose circulating in your blood that you can use for energy. Humans require a lot of energy; even our basal metabolic rate—the energy needed for basic functions like walking, breathing, and staying upright—demands a significant amount.

If you have more glucose than your body needs, though, your body stores it in the form of glycogen, the storage form of glucose. You have glycogen stored in your muscles and your liver.

Let's say you don't eat for a while. Maybe you go outside for a walk. Your body will recognize it needs more energy and will release some of this stored glycogen. If you're walking, it will release it from the muscles.

If you exhaust all the glycogen stored in the muscles, it will release it from the liver. You basically have different energy tanks you're using to power yourself. The glycogen tank is very, very small compared to your fat storage tank. For example, one pound of stored fat can provide the average person with almost two days of energy.

If we exert ourselves enough to empty the glycogen tank (think hours upon hours of exercise), our body goes to the fat storage tank. This presents us with a few options when it comes to losing weight.

Either we need to go for periods without eating—usually, around sixteen hours to twenty-four—or we need to increase our activity levels to the point where we can deplete that glycogen tank faster.

Knowing when to eat is useful because it helps us understand our bodies better. Ten thousand years ago, we didn't have Costco or Sam's Club. There was no refrigerator, and not even a corner store; humans had to deal with feast-or-famine conditions. If we didn't have food for a day, our body had to figure out a way to store things so when it needed something, it could access it.

That's basically how we ended up with our insulin mechanism and body fat.

Body fat is our long-term energy storage system. Let's say you didn't eat for a day and you've run out of all your glycogen reserves. Your body switches and begins to burn fat for energy.

On the other hand, if you've eaten a big meal, one that gives you more energy than you need, your body switches to fat storage. It's constantly trying to figure out which energy source is the best to use at the moment; our bodies have the ability to burn both glucose and fat.

In general, when we're looking at weight loss, we're trying to help the body get into that fat storage tank and burn more of what's there. Most people could go for days without eating because their bodies would continuously provide them with energy by breaking down their extra fat and using it for energy.

One strategy used for insulin-resistant people is to employ intermittent fasting. Intermittent fasting means we go without any calories intentionally for a period of time so we can get better at burning what we've stored in that fat storage tank. While calories in and calories out does matter, intermittent fasting is a way we can harness the power of our ancestral physiology and help maintain control over our insulin and blood sugar responses. I'll talk about that more in the next section.

The Three Levers

Dr. Peter Attia has defined three levers people can use when manipulating their diets. I agree these are the three main strategies at work when trying to make meaningful changes in our nutrition. These levers are:

- Timing: Paying attention to or dictating when you eat and when you don't.
- Quantity: Managing the total volume of food you consume in a day.
- Composition: Adjusting the types of food you eat.

Let's look at each of these in more detail.

Timing

Timing refers to when you're eating and when you're not eating. Creating a window of fasting for some people, even if it's just overnight, can be a huge step forward. A twelve-hour window is a great place to begin if you're just getting started with intermittent fasting. And it's not that hard to do!

If you go to bed at 10:00 or 10:30 p.m., you'll have your last meal two hours before bed. It's not that hard to hold off on breakfast until 8:00 a.m. the next day, and that gives you your twelve-hour window.

This is very much in line with how your body would have done this ancestrally. We wouldn't have been eating at 10:00

p.m. each night; we'd be sleeping! As an added benefit, creating a little time without eating before we sleep will help us massively in that area, as we learned back in Chapter 7.

When we talk about breaking a fast, we should also be specific about what foods or drinks will do that. If you have any fluids that don't include calories, like herbal tea, black coffee, water, or even a squeeze of lemon water, that's fine; those don't give your body any calories to process. If you put milk or cream in your coffee, that would be enough to break your fast from the purest perspective. It would signal to your body that you're getting ready to eat again.

For people struggling with extra body fat and trying to improve their body composition, intermittent fasting can be effective. If you can do it about three days a week, the magic number you want to work up to is sixteen hours.

Depending on your activity level, your body has enough stored glycogen to last anywhere from fourteen to twenty hours. If you can burn through that, your body will switch to a fat-burning mode. Not only does this help with fat loss, but it's great for those with insulin resistance.

If you're trying to get to a sixteen-hour window, you can skip breakfast intentionally, eat a normal lunch, normal dinner, and possibly even a small snack after dinner, and then not eat anything after that for the next sixteen hours. A lot of people have had success with this because it's an easy way to improve your metabolic health.

But isn't breakfast the most important meal of the day?

You may not know that statement was originally coined by the breakfast cereal companies. The first meal of the day is still your most important meal because it sets the tone for your day—but it doesn't have to be "breakfast" in the sense of strictly eating your first meal in the morning. It could be lunch.

If the first thing you eat in the morning consists of toast, cereal, muffins, pancakes, and orange juice, you're basically creating a large insulin response first thing in the day. Whenever we consume a high-carbohydrate breakfast, our body has no choice but to match the level of glucose. It'll try to bring your blood sugar back into the normal range by secreting insulin. The more often you do these big swings, the more susceptible you'll be to Type 2 diabetes.

As your blood sugar swings back down, your brain will start to crave things that will bring the sugar back up. Our goal is to eliminate those big swings.

Besides that, these big-sugar swings aren't pleasant to deal with in the short term. They create energy and mood swings as your blood sugar goes up and down. This is where being "hangry" comes from, as well as your afternoon slump. If you make your first meal savory instead of sweet, it'll have a huge influence on how your whole day goes.

If you're fit, then maybe intermittent fasting isn't something you have to consider. Most of the patients I see, however, are trying to manage inflammation and improve their blood sugar. We want metabolic improvement, so intermittent fasting is a good answer. Again, you don't have to do this every day! Three times a week of this sixteen-hour practice will work.

Quantity

Our second lever is how much food you consume. Once again, if you're trying to make a change in your body composition or weight, we'd be talking about the total volume you'd eat in a normal day. This also encompasses the main theory of weight loss, which is "calories in, calories out." If you decrease your caloric intake for a certain number of weeks or months, you will typically lose weight.

That being said, if you decrease your caloric intake too much and for too long, it will slow down your metabolic rate. Your metabolism works like a thermostat; we all burn a certain number of calories when at rest, which is called our basal metabolic rate. Over time, people plateau. Their bodies say, "Okay, well, I don't have as much food, so I better slow things down so I can survive better long-term." That makes it easier for people to yo-yo back up to higher weights: When your basal metabolic rate is low, if you increase your caloric intake, then you start storing those excess calories as body fat again.

Composition

The third lever involves what you eat. All the strategies we've talked about in this chapter and beyond—keto, paleo, low-carb, vegetarian, vegan, carnivore—are ways we manipulate what foods we eat. They can have a dramatic effect on how people feel, but also on their body composition and metabolism.

There's plenty to focus on here, but it's important to select what works best for you. To reiterate, what we've found from all these studies is that pretty much anything is better than the standard North American diet.

When you're ready to implement the levers, start by cutting out certain foods. It's easy to get overwhelmed if you change too many things at once. We're trying to simplify this by focusing on one lever at a time to help you gain the momentum you need.

If one lever stops working, you may find you have to use another set of strategies to keep the body moving in the direction you want it to go. Let's say someone's done caloric restriction for a long time, lost twenty pounds, and plateaued; what can they do? Well, if they change what they eat on that same number of calories, changing the composition of them, that's a lever that might spur the body into action.

For example you might want to increase your protein intake. Not only will you feel full for longer, but it will also help you with those sweet cravings and make it easier to sustain over the long term. Alternatively, you could decrease your calories from carbohydrates and increase your fat calories to the point of putting your body into a state of ketosis—where your body's main source of energy is by turning fat into ketones for energy. For a lot of people, these strategies work very well in conjunction with each other.

It's possible that a longer fast may jumpstart things, but always check with your healthcare provider first. If you're interested in reading more about this, check out the work of Dr. Valter Longo.

For those who measure not just weight, but body fat percentage versus lean tissue, intermittent fasting can be of great help...but still within limits. Too much and you can develop changes in your thyroid. Your metabolism slows down and can affect your mood; you might feel depressed and have less energy. Implementing intermittent fasting for the short term is much easier to manage and reduces all those risks.

As someone who is at risk for insulin resistance, I've personally used these levers to help me manage my blood sugar levels.

I had my A1C done fifteen years ago. My naturopath told me my numbers were way too high for me based on my goals and family history—it was 5.7. I cut out juices from my diet and made some pretty drastic changes. I started cutting down on grains, and my blood sugar went down in about three months. I hadn't checked it until 2020, when I was investigating my Vitamin D3 intake. Back then, it was at 5.5. That's decent—not amazing, but not anything to worry about.

These past few years, I've been doing intermittent fasting, eating low carb, and nothing that feels too restrictive or extreme, and I've managed to get my A1C down to 4.6. That's literally a full point down within a few years of me implementing these things.

I'm not a special case. My father had diabetes. The rest of my family struggles with their weight. I'm definitely not the fittest person in the room. But through using these three levers, I've been able to manage my own blood sugar and get my metabolic health where it needs to be. As my patients apply these things, some of them are able to reduce their dependence on levels of their medication for Type 2 diabetes. If you use these levers effectively, you can help your physiology do what it's naturally supposed to do.

Good Goals

Everyone seems to focus on weight loss as a goal, but the focus should be on creating a long-term habit rather than the outcome of that habit. Sometimes it's nice to have a number in mind, but that can also be really frustrating. What often happens is they'll lose weight at the start of a new diet, but then things will slow down. That's discouraging.

I don't like the scale as the only metric to measure success because people may emotionally go up and down as their weight fluctuates. That's a dangerous cycle to sign up for. While being aware of your weight can be helpful, a good substitute for this can be measuring your waist size. It's a simple alternative and one of the methods used to determine metabolic syndrome. For men, aim for under forty inches, and for women, aim for under thirty-five inches.

What about using body-mass index (BMI) as a metric? BMI is just not a good system to use. You can have someone who's fairly fit and not very tall, but their BMI puts them in the obese range. That's not an accurate representation of their health! They're just not tall.

Most guys want to get back to the weight they were when they felt their best; for many, that's high school or college. They have a direct line to get there. Women who are still having their menstrual cycles, however, experience more weight fluctuations. I've seen water retention that can add up to four pounds a day! Depending on where they are in their cycle, their weight could oscillate by that much. That's an emotional nightmare if weight is the only goal you're focusing on.

That's why I encourage my patients not only to focus on an outcome like waist size but to focus on implementing the habits and systems that will create the result they are looking for. Ask yourself, "What can I do each day that's different?" I always want to give some kind of target for my patients' brains to aim at; by taking the focus off the scales, we can implement other changes, like lifting weights and drinking more water, where we might not see the scales change at all, but make changes in body composition. The old saying, "A pound of muscle weighs more than a pound of fat" is not true. A pound is a pound is a pound. What is true is muscle is more metabolically active than fat, so your goal should be to increase your lean muscle mass and decrease your body fat. Understand that your weight might not change on the scale, but your waist-size may go down. Getting rid of belly fat is a great step to better metabolic health and decreasing your risk of all causes of mortality.

If I had to choose one metric for people to make the effort to change, it would be body fat percentage. Depending on your age and sex, your goal range will be different. Men have lower ranges of body fat than women do. Ideal ranges for men would be 12-20 percent and for women 20-30 percent. The older we get, the more those ranges increase. Don't obsess about the number. Again, focus on the habits and systems that would consistently bring you results, and be consistent. Change takes time.

That being said, it's not easy for the average person to measure their body fat percentage accurately. While some scales offer estimates, getting a precise measurement typically requires specialized equipment like a DEXA scan or consulting a professional, which can be cumbersome and expensive. But if it's possible for you, I highly recommend it.

I often ask the groups I coach, "What's the most destructive habit you have in terms of achieving your goal? What's going to hold you back the most?" For some, it's late-night eating. For others, it's snacking too much, or too much sugar. Most people have a general idea of what they need to do; they just don't know the specifics, or what levers they can use to get where they want to go. In the last ten years, intermittent fasting has gained a lot of traction because people have found it's an easy way to manage food without having to be rigorous with all their food tracking and calorie counting. I don't think this will be a trendy thing; it's going to be something people understand as a legitimate and meaningful way to manage their insulin response and lose dangerous abdominal fat.

When working on these goals, perhaps the biggest gift you can give yourself is time. If you set a goal for something that's too big or intimidating, like one hundred pounds, that might be too far out of reach for the average person, at least immediately. Could someone do it? Absolutely. What typically happens, however, is the weight loss starts taking a long time; they're focused on the one hundred pounds and not celebrating the ten-, twenty-, and thirty-pound losses that it takes to get there. They get distracted...and then they lose interest.

To help you pick a smart goal, one that has long-term potential, but is also achievable in the interim:

1. **Think back to your long-term vision:** How do you want to look in twenty years? What's a good first step toward that? For some people, that may be an interim weight loss goal and adopting the habits that need to shift to get you there.

2. **Identify as a healthy person:** What would the healthiest version of yourself do daily? How would they grocery shop? How would they prepare food?

Game Changers—Putting All This to Good Use

Now that you understand the dynamics of your food choices, remember you have the power to change what you eat. To get started, let's take a look at some of the steps we covered in this chapter a little more closely:

1. **Identify Your Individual Needs:** Understand your body's unique requirements and responses to food.

Experiment and observe to tailor your diet for optimal health.

2. **Reduce Processed Foods:** Cut back on processed foods containing chemicals, sugars, and industrial seed oils that cause inflammation and long-term health issues.

3. **Set Short-Term Dietary Goals:** Establish clear, short-term goals to reduce decision fatigue and maintain consistency in your eating habits.

4. **Prioritize Whole Foods:** Focus on fresh, whole foods found in the perimeter of grocery stores. Choose organic options and clean sources of animal protein like grass-fed beef and wild-caught seafood.

5. **Read Labels and Reduce Added Sugars:** Check food labels for hidden sugars and prioritize foods with higher protein content. Limit added sugars and choose foods with minimal processing.

6. **Protein Intake:** Aim for 0.7 to 0.8 grams of protein per pound of body weight. Choose high-quality protein sources and monitor intake for weight management or muscle maintenance.

7. **Carbohydrate Selection:** Get carbohydrates primarily from vegetables and fruits with lower glycemic index. Consider individual factors when determining carbohydrate intake and prioritize nutrient-dense options.

8. **Healthy Fat Consumption:** Incorporate healthy fats like fatty fish, olive oil, and avocados into your diet. Prioritize Omega-3-rich foods and supplement if needed.

9. **Hydration:** Drink half your body weight in ounces of water daily, adjusting for caffeine intake by adding extra water. Consider adding salt to maintain electrolyte balance, especially on a low-carb diet.

10. **Natural Sweeteners:** Experiment with natural sweeteners like stevia, erythritol, or monk fruit to satisfy sweet cravings without spiking blood sugar levels if you're feeling intimidated about cutting out sugars.

11. **Physical Activity:** Incorporate regular physical activity like walking after meals to stabilize blood sugar levels and utilize stored glycogen for energy.

12. **Intermittent Fasting:** Consider intermittent fasting to improve insulin sensitivity and promote fat burning by allowing the body to access stored energy reserves.

13. **Utilize the Three Levers:** Implement one lever at a time (timing, quantity, or composition) to gain momentum and switch them up if you hit a plateau.

By implementing these steps, you can create changes to your environment that support your health goals without relying solely on willpower. And when times get tough, don't forget to stay connected to your *why*. Make sure to check out my YouTube channel if you need a visual explanation to these concepts.

I'll help you further define your action steps, along with the Two-Week Food Challenge, in Chapter 11.

CHAPTER 10

Pillar Six:
Stress Management

One of my clients, Catherine, was referred to me by an acupuncturist. Unfortunately, Catherine, who is in her early seventies, has multi-level joint pain and pain in her knuckles, hips, neck, and jaw. Her doctor basically told her she has arthritis in all of these joints. Thanks to the acupuncturist, she found some relief through dietary changes and came to me to help sort out the other stuff.

We were able to get most of the other pain under control. Then her husband was diagnosed with cancer. All of a sudden, the symptoms we'd managed for some time came roaring back. What happened?

I've seen this occur, especially in my patients with arthritis. Usually, it occurs when they make a small dietary change— like sneaking something they know they are sensitive to into a meal—and they experience a flare in their joints.

Suspecting Catherine did something like that, I asked her if her eating habits had changed; she said no.

I went through the rest of my health checklist, through all the other nutritional culprits that might cause a flare-up for her. Still nothing. I asked how she was sleeping. It was the same as before.

Across every axis of health I could name, everything was the same for her. Catherine hadn't changed anything in her diet or what we were working on at the clinic, and she was still seeing her acupuncturist. The only thing different in her life was her husband's diagnosis and all of his appointments and radiation treatments, which she attended.

Understandably, she was an emotional mess for months. When all that settled down and her husband got a cleaner bill of health, Catherine's symptoms eased. The flare-up passed.

In short, she had been stressed out. Even though she had been doing everything right, her health problems had started to come back.

That's the power of stress.

Good Stress vs. Bad Stress

It's impossible to exist in the modern world without running into stress. It's everywhere; in the workplace, in our personal lives, or joked about online. Just as we can't go through life without facing challenges, we also can't go through life without occasionally dealing with stressful situations.

That being said, there's good stress and bad stress.

The most common good stressor is working out. Lifting weights puts a demand on your body, but it's a positive stressor because it spurs your body to adapt in a way that makes it stronger. Yes, we may be tearing down tissues in the moment, but they build back tougher.

Weight-bearing exercise is another good one and a prime example is walking. When you walk, you put stress on your bones, but ultimately, that's good because it helps you maintain your bone density. Astronauts often experience this as a problem when they return to Earth: they're so used to living without gravity that they need specific exercises to help rebuild their bone density. When I work out, even though it is a demand on my body, I think of it as a good stressor because it's something I genuinely enjoy doing. It gives me the energy to handle the rest of my day, even as I'm putting effort into it.

In short, good stressors help us better handle the regular things we have to do. Doing them rewards you in some way down the line.

A bad stressor is something that's more than your body can accommodate. In the physical world, it might look like working out too much or doing excessive physical labor. If it's too hard for you, your body won't be able to recover normally. Your muscle tissue gets torn down too much and you might create an injury.

However, what happens for too many people is the demands they place on their bodies are greater than what they're giving back to them. Think about your body like a bank account. Throughout the day, the actions you take act as deposits and withdrawals. It's very easy not to be intentional and to keep making all those withdrawals. Work stress, family stress, money stress—all those things take energy out of your body's account without putting anything back in. I'm not saying we shouldn't have those things in our lives, like fulfilling work, a loving family, and a stable income; rather, we need to create counterbalances to deal with the stress they bring.

Different people also handle stress differently. What I do might be very stressful for someone else. A large part of handling stress is knowing where your own stress tolerances lie.

The important thing to remember is we're not supposed to live in a constant state of stress. That's how we become overwhelmed, and I see many people who feel that way in my practice. I try to focus on what I can do to respond to the stressors around me rather than trying to change them. Sometimes, it's just a difference of perspective.

We're not supposed to live in a constant state of stress, but we're also not supposed to live without it. Remember from the last chapter that our bodies are perfectly happy existing in a feast-or-famine state; we have mechanisms in place in case we don't have food. Just like our bodies have adapted to states of feast or famine, we have adapted to dealing with different kinds of stress.

Part of how we do that is through rest. If you're an ancient human and you've been walking around and hunting for food all day, your body is going to need a certain level of rest. Sleep is the counterbalance to physical activity, one of the many checks and balances your body has to keep everything functioning smoothly.

What the body doesn't have is a good way to deal with stress coming at it from multiple places. That's where your perception and insight are so vital. If you perceive your work environment or family to be stressful, if you have a tough financial situation you're going through, then your body will pick up on that. It won't operate at full capacity because it wants to be able to deal with whatever stress you feel is imminent.

Much of my work involves helping people build more capacity to take on the things they want to, the things that feel more fulfilling. I've also done that in my own life; I can take on more ambitious projects because I've put more deposits into my health and well-being. This motivated me to come up with the pillars included in this book.

It's like having a cup. There's only so much stress you can pour into the cup before it overflows and you feel overwhelmed. By taking care of your health, you can increase the capacity of your cup. You can deal with more stress. When you start asking more from yourself and finding you have the ability to deliver on that, life gets really interesting.

Some of these things are also cumulative. I'm working out the same way I was ten years ago; that hasn't changed. I'm doing some biohacking things now that I wasn't doing then. (Biohacking is trying to enhance your biology through supplements and lifestyle changes.) My wife and I built our own building, we ran a business, and I coached two sports teams.

At the peak of our busyness, our kids had about twenty sporting events per week between them, and that's not an exaggeration. Some days I went from seeing patients to my workout, then from my workout to a team meeting, then home to get my kids organized. I would make them supper, and then it was off to hockey, volleyball, basketball, and/or baseball! That's a lot!

I often remind myself that I have made these choices, so it's not stressful for me, but it's easy to see how it could be overwhelming for someone else. The difference is I've structured my life around building up my own capacity to support this kind of life. You can do that, too, and that's what we'll spend this chapter exploring: How do you get a bigger cup?

Chronic Stress

We know from previous chapters that our body has two parts to the autonomic nervous system, the sympathetic and the parasympathetic. We need both. The parasympathetic is responsible for our rest and digest mechanism and the sympathetic is our fight-or-flight. We still encounter scary situations we want to get out of quickly, but sometimes we find ourselves in interactions that trigger our stress response but really shouldn't.

Back in the days of our ancestors, we might have had to run away from saber-toothed tigers or other natural dangers. These days, that part of our brain sometimes gets activated when we get in fights with our kids, experience bad drivers on the road, realize we're not in love with our jobs, or some other stressor. All day long, we create this sympathetic response to our problems, and then we make bad decisions...often with food.

What's actually happening in our body is a hormonal response. Certain chemicals get released into the bloodstream when we're stressed, like cortisol and epinephrine. These make our blood pressure and heart rate increase. They are there to help us run away or fight whatever we feel is threatening us. Having these chemicals in our blood long-term isn't healthy, however.

When your sympathetic nervous system is triggered, your body doesn't process food the same way as when you're in the parasympathetic state. In the sympathetic state, blood flows away from the organs in your digestive tract and toward the extremities. If you're constantly stressed out, it can affect things like digestion and elimination; it can literally give you bowel problems, anything from IBS to constipation. Getting a better handle on your nervous system can help you improve your digestive health and even how sensitive you are to insulin.

Remember our chapter on sleep? Stress, as you've probably experienced, also affects how we sleep. Our sleep reflects the kind of day we've had. If we've received a ton of stress hormones during the day, it can affect whether we get to sleep or have trouble staying asleep. So many people have these sleep problems, which, in turn, affect everything else about their health.

Mentally, stress can manifest as having the same thoughts on a loop over and over again. Many people have the same stressful thoughts on repeat all day long. Listen to your self-talk. Is it how you'd talk to a friend? Or is it something else?

Anytime I'm starting to feel a bit stressed, I'll remind myself that I've chosen all of these things. There were some days when I had six or seven "kid things" I had to take care of as a parent. This could be overwhelming, but it's also stuff I know makes my kids happy. So, it makes me happy too, even if it takes some effect on my part to make it happen.

My wife and I voluntarily had kids. We knew it would happen that we'd get busy. When I reaffirm to myself that I chose this and I'm doing what I want to be doing, I feel much happier. I'm happy to support them.

Again, this is why our frameworks of perception are so important. Often when I talk to people who are overwhelmed, they have looping stressful thoughts. That is where self-talk comes into play.

I often ask people what their most dominant thought is. You can learn a lot from somebody by finding out what they tell themselves on repeat or having them write it down. What do you stress about the most?

Once you know what that is, you can begin to address it.

Responses to Stress

Something many of my habitually stressed-out patients have in common is a tightness in their upper backs, specifically around their trapezius muscles. These muscles, your "traps," are between your neck and shoulders, and for many people, they're perennially stiff. That tightness can be due to a stress response; muscles become tight after repeated usage. If you're tensing up your shoulders a lot because you're frequently stressed out, then you're going to have tight shoulders.

Other patients get tremendous headaches or clench and grind their teeth at night. These are all manifestations of the emotional things that affect them, whether it's based in anger, fear, or frustration. How your parents handled stress when you were growing up will also influence how you handle stress as an adult. It's a learned behavior we picked up as kids.

The most important thing to understand about stress is the accumulated effect it has on the body. Going back to our analogy of the cup, we're trying to contain this accumulated stress the best we can. If it's one isolated event stressing us out, generally that's not too difficult for us to manage. Sometimes things will go wrong, and that's just a part of life. Each of us has a threshold, however, where enough stressful things add up to become truly difficult for us to manage.

Scientists have posited that one of the differences between humans and animals can be boiled down to the stress response. Take a deer in a forest. When it hears the approach of a predator, the deer bolts, running through the trees to safety. Five minutes later, that same deer is back to eating grass. The deer isn't thinking about what was chasing it before, or even worried about the predator anymore. With humans, we have these events that happen in our life as well as our brain's perception of them. We can either let the event go, or we can choose to hang on to it and allow it to persist and continue to influence us. That decision is up to us, and what we choose will affect our bodies.

At the end of the day, our body will either help us reach our goals in life or present one of the biggest obstacles we have to overcome. I have patients who sleep decently, exercise, take supplements, and eat well—but this whole mental piece is where they fall apart. They will come into my office with this emotional history that's affecting them physically; that's part of what we have to sort through because it's influencing their ability to change their health.

Your perception of your life is a significant piece of the puzzle. In fact, it's so important that I made it one of my pillars of health.

I'm not a counselor or psychiatrist, but even looking at this from purely a sports and health lens, the influence is obvious. I can't speak to some of the wounds you may be dealing with, but I can tell you that working on your internal wellbeing will make you a better and healthier person. We retain trauma at the cellular level; it's worth the time and effort to heal that.

In my practice, I always wonder why some techniques and protocols work for certain people and not others. One main differentiating factor I've found has been stress. Often, I've discovered underlying stuff was at work, or perhaps their home life was getting to be too much, or they were settling into new responsibilities with something else. Acknowledging that and working to address it can make a real difference in getting results.

My goal is to find ways to get people where they want to go. The more I look at their stress response, the more I see it having a massive impact on my patients' well-being. Some people don't want to talk about these things. However, when people share with me what's happened to them, I can see where their body is holding on to that emotional pain. Some clients don't share emotional information with me, but I can still tell they're holding on to something somewhere.

If this discussion resonates with you, I highly encourage you to work through your emotional stressors. Whether that's seeing a mental health professional, taking up a meditative or journaling practice, breathwork, or a multitude of other options, addressing past wounds will help build your physical health and give you more influence over your nervous system.

Breath

The human body is not designed to move at a hundred miles an hour all the time. If we find ourselves living in a constantly activated, stressed-out state, we need to find ways to get back to our parasympathetic nervous system, out of the panic and back into calm. Breathing with intention is a great path back to that.

Some ways to breathe calm us down…and other ways do the opposite. We can breathe through our nose and our mouth, and the airway we use matters.

As a chiropractor, I pick up on people's movements. When someone's lying face-down on the table and I ask them to take a deep breath, I can literally see which part of their body is generating the breath. If they're breathing through their mouth and I ask them to take deep breaths, I can see them not using their diaphragm. Initially their breaths will be shallow, but If I want them to relax, I will instruct them to breathe deeply through their belly.

We know that when our bodies are under stress, we tend to breathe through our mouths. This engages accessory breathing muscles along the front of the neck. When I have a patient who primarily uses their mouth to breathe, these muscles along the front of their neck will feel like ropes. They've been using their accessory muscles to breathe so much that those muscles have gotten tight.

Breathing from our chest versus breathing from our belly is also another huge factor. If I want someone to relax, not only will I tell them to breathe through their nose, but I'll tell them to breathe from their belly. This encourages them to take a truly deep breath by engaging their diaphragm. Studies have shown that if you do diaphragmatic breathing for a few minutes, you'll reduce your cortisol (a stress hormone) levels.

Another benefit of nasal breathing is it filters the air entering our bodies. It also helps us generate more nitric oxide, a vasodilator. This means it helps blood vessels relax or dilate. As you can see, different breathing patterns can help ground our bodies and reduce chemical stressors in our circulatory system.

Chronic stress, from a cardiovascular perspective, is not good for us. It increases our blood pressure as well as our heart rate. We know those two things increasing in tandem are detrimental to heart health. If your body's "normal" state becomes one of chronic stress, you'll see an increased risk of heart attack, thanks to higher blood pressure's impact on your blood vessels.

Because breathwork can have such a profound influence on lowering stress levels, people from many demanding walks of life have implemented it. One of the most notable examples is the Navy SEALs, who popularized box breathing.

Obviously, being a Navy SEAL is a very stressful job. You have to be prepared for anything at the drop of a hat. They found that if you can control your breathing, you can also gain control of your emotions and keep cool in a high-pressure situation.

Box breathing is a four-second cycle. You breathe in for four seconds, hold that breath for four seconds, breathe out for four seconds, and then hold that out for four seconds. Then, you repeat it as many times as you need to, following the lines of the box. If you do box breathing for two minutes, it will reduce your cortisol.

I run my life by appointments—makes sense, right? People call my office all the time in traffic, apologizing and frantically telling me there is heavy traffic so they'll be late today. The very first thing I have them do when they get to the clinic is to slow down their breathing. If I don't do this, I know the patient won't get the most out of their adjustment. Their body will be too wound up for anything I do to have an effect. If I have them do box breathing for two minutes, it can be the game-changer between a mediocre appointment and one that makes a big difference.

A regular meditation practice is also something I encourage. If you're interested in getting started with meditation or breathwork, I have videos on them that you can view on my YouTube channel, Dr. Jason Plotsky, along with additional information there.

I especially recommend Wim Hof for breathwork. A Dutch extreme athlete, motivational speaker, and founder of the Wim Hof Method®, Hof has set a number of records for cold exposure, running through the desert without water, and climbing mountains without a shirt. He has led a fascinating life, and I'm such a big fan I recorded my own version of this breathing method that you can view for free on my YouTube channel.

The Wim Hof Method is basically thirty big breaths in, to hyperoxygenate your body, then a breath hold. This is to your own comfort level; if you don't feel like you can hold your breath very long, then don't. What happens over time is you can train your body to do longer and longer breath holds. This is another example of a good, controlled stress.

I've been doing Wim Hof's training for some time, and I've recently been able to crack two minutes for holding my breath. I would not have been able to do that without his techniques.

Part of why I've been so focused on breath is you can change your blood chemistry via your breathwork. Wim Hof is also very knowledgeable, and a great resource on this. He calls his thirty-second-breath-and-hold method alkalizing.

Hof's cold exposure work may be what he's most famous for, and he says that everything comes back to training. Your breathwork is training you to hold your breath longer. When you hop in a cold shower, you can train yourself to stay in there longer by training your body not to panic and to breathe instead.

It's honestly amazing what you can change with a little intentionality.

Other people have postulated that if your cells aren't getting enough oxygen, they can't live as well or as long. Breathwork helps us on so many levels to stay and remain healthy, both physically and mentally. Often, meditation may look like sitting with your legs crossed, but it doesn't have to be. For me, meditation can also be walking with my dog in nature or playing catch with my boys. Whatever gets your brain to slow down and be in the present moment is good for your nervous system.

Meditation as a Practice

I could talk about the benefits of meditation for days. A few years ago, I took a weeklong course with Dr. Joe Dispenza, one of the world's leading experts in meditation. Studies on the effects of a single weekend meditation show a change in people's stress response after just a few days.

Personally, I use meditation as much as I can. I've found it to be incredibly effective, even if it's in small increments like just before going to bed or immediately when I wake up. For patients new to this side of health, I usually start off by recommending breathing exercises because they're easier to incorporate. You can do them sitting in your car, breathing through your nose, diaphragmatically, and trying box breathing. Breathwork requires nothing more than your willingness to give it a try. The two recordings on my site are seven and ten minutes long, so they are easy for most people to incorporate into their day.

Remember Catherine from the beginning of the chapter? She became a fan of Dr. Dispenza's meditations. I had done a few guided ones I really liked and I recommended them to her, so she started there. I've found I've had the most success with guided meditations, having someone else walk me through the process of relaxing, so those tend to be what I prefer. With a guide, my brain has something to focus on.

Catherine did the guided meditations for about twenty to thirty minutes each day, and that really helped. We worked through a checklist together as we addressed her stress. Breathwork wasn't cutting it for her...until she discovered the meditations. They became her game-changer.

Even now, sometimes she'll come into my office stressed and I'll run through the checklist of things that might be wrong. She usually eats, sleeps, and exercises well. When I ask if she's been meditating during those stressful weeks, she'll look up and say no. Then I tell her that's her homework. We know meditation is what moves the needle for her overall health, even when she's doing everything else right.

Herbal Supplements for Stress

A lot of conversation has ensued around different herbal curatives for stress. Most herbs are fine for most people, but a few need to be used with more caution, depending on individual health conditions.

For instance, ashwagandha is effective for managing stress and reducing cortisol, but it can also lower blood pressure. If you're on blood pressure medication, consult your healthcare provider or pharmacist before using it. Other safe and helpful options include L-theanine and GABA, which also support stress reduction by decreasing cortisol and improving the relaxation response.

With so many herbal options available, finding the right one can make a significant difference in managing stress. However, be sure to check with your healthcare provider to ensure they are safe for you.

Addressing Emotional Wounds

In general, I've found that people's problems tend to fall into one of three categories: physical, chemical, or mental/emotional. It's part of my job to help people figure out which. Because what I do in my practice is physical, that's always where I start. It's also not too difficult to give people some homework on the chemical side—we've already talked about simple ways to start changing that for the better with supplements and better nutrition.

I constantly feel like mental health is an underserved and understated part of our overall health. It's overlooked as a cause of problems that people often face and have to face alone. In Canada, one in three people will experience some type of mental health stressor in their life.

The fact is people can't just remove emotional stressors from their lives. I have a client who, even though she comes to her appointments regularly, remains worried that she can't just quit her job or leave her family. She may not even want to do either of those things! But she needs a way to better endure that added pressure. Once you have kids, you can't go back to not having kids. You have to find a way to adapt to your new reality.

You have to get creative in teaching your body how to deal with your life.

Some things you may not be able to change like work, finances, or family. That doesn't mean you can't improve your circumstances. To begin making those improvements, I can't recommend enough breathwork, meditation, and thoughtful journaling.

I can recommend a few apps, both free and paid, if you're interested in getting started in a mindfulness practice. Calm, Headspace, and Insight Timer are some popular ones.

Again, my YouTube channel, Dr. Jason Plotsky, has guided breath work available if you want to check them out. Whatever you decide to do, beginning and taking the first step toward better mental and emotional health is a big move.

The End of the Pillars

With this chapter, we've reached the end of my six pillars of health—my checklist of the most important aspects of our health.

Ultimately, though, you won't be able to optimize these pillars without commitment. Lifestyle changes aren't easy, and to implement them, as we'll discuss in the next chapter, you'll need a strong why. What is driving you to improve your health? What will you turn to for leverage when you need to retain focus on this longer goal? Anybody can do something for a weekend; a week is harder, but still doable. If you can follow these principles for twenty-one days, I want to know what's driving you to get to day twenty-two.

There's a difference between discipline and motivation. Discipline is the ability to do hard things when you don't want to do them. You do the workout when you're already tired. You go grocery shopping for clean food even when all you really want to do is eat out. Motivation will come and go, but discipline is what will help you achieve your long-term goals.

Every time you keep a promise to yourself, you build your self-esteem. As you get better and better at keeping those promises, you can take on harder and harder things. You can challenge yourself more because you believe in your ability to meet your goals. The world becomes your oyster.

I'll be honest with you: A lot of this stuff is hard, and sometimes that means we will try hard and still end up failing. Get up and try again. Remember, your body is designed to be healthy, and your job is to figure out how to unlock its true healing powers.

CHAPTER 11

Implementation

It's easy to get overwhelmed by all this new information. That's okay! Don't feel like you need to change thirty things in your life immediately. Your goals for the long term can be ambitious (and I encourage that), but to be effective, they need to be implemented properly.

You need sustainable change, goals that can be broken down into small, manageable steps. In this final chapter, you'll see how to do just that and put everything you've learned into practice.

Here's my challenge for you: What can you do in three years to dramatically change your health? Patience is necessary here; we won't be able to achieve these goals overnight. What's your mental image of where you want to be not just next week, but in the next five, ten, or twenty years? Do you want to be in your late seventies and traveling the world? Don't say you're going to "wing it"—that will probably end up with you in a nursing home being looked after by somebody else for the last few years of your life.

Everyone is good at procrastinating. Few people are good at acting when urgency doesn't compel them to. Having a clear goal can help instill that urgency in us. I explain this to people as a choice between doing the difficult thing now or dealing with the difficult thing later. It's hard to change your diet and exercise, but it's also hard living with cancer and diabetes. So, pick your hard.

Sometimes people forget that. It's easy to think that everything's going to magically be okay and then be surprised when it's not. Then they get overwhelmed when they see how hard things can be when they're not healthy.

Don't let that be you. The choices you make now will dictate your health later. And I know it's hard to change these things, believe me. But if you want a specific outcome and can clearly visualize what you want your life to look like in the future, you'll likely be willing to put up with doing the hard things now.

After reading through these pillars, you probably already know which one you should spend the most time working on. To help you get started, I've created a checklist for you to use according to your level, Level One or Level Two.

Level One Checklist

Consider yourself a Level One? Here are five steps to get you started:

1. Drink more water.

Water intake is where I start with almost everyone. Drink half of your body weight in ounces over the course of a day.

Consider adding a quality electrolyte or simply a small amount of salt like Redmond sea salt to your water.

2. Incorporate three supplements.

You can check with your health practitioner to see which supplements you would benefit most from adding, but Vitamin D3 (with K2), magnesium, and Omega-3s like fish oil are great places to start.

3. Start moving.

Consider the amount of exercise you get each week. Are you getting the recommended 150 minutes? If it seems intimidating, start small and grow from there. Ask yourself how you can add ten, fifteen, or twenty minutes of something simple like walking per day.

4. Avoid processed foods.

This is often a difficult step for Level One individuals. You don't need to start a specific diet, simply limit (and eventually eliminate) as many fast foods, packaged foods, and as much added sugar as possible. An easy way to start? Start perimeter shopping at the grocery store and focus on incorporating mostly single ingredient foods.

5. Work on your sleep.

As a Level One, just focus on two things: getting to bed by 11 p.m. and reducing your blue light exposure (turn off your devices!) one hour before bed. When your sleep improves, so will almost every other aspect of your life.

If every one of my patients did these five things, they would transform their health. For some people, however, this isn't enough; some people need more specific diet recommendations and more rigorous exercise. If we want to slow down aging, for example, walking isn't enough on its own. We have to engage muscles, build strength, and work on resistance training, which we focus on in Level Two.

But for Level Ones, this strategy will at least keep down inflammation and get you headed down the right path. If your goal is to prevent metabolic syndrome and ultimately the Big Four from happening for as long as you can, then this is a great start.

Level Two Checklist

If the things on the Level One checklist sound easy to you, or you're already doing them in your daily life, then you may be ready for Level Two. Here's where to start:

1. Start resistance training.

Resistance training is the next step in the exercise pyramid after you implement more basic movement like walking. It's also where a lot of people get stuck. If you read "resistance training" and suddenly got nervous, try to shift your mindset.

Resistance training simply means moving against resistance. It could be in the form of bodyweight exercises, using bands, going to the gym to lift weights, or even swimming. Moving against resistance will help with your bone density and muscle health. (It will help you build more lean tissue—or at least maintain what you have—which is important as you age.) Aim for two sessions a week. It will give you a lot of bang for your buck, so don't skip it.

2. Add more supplements.

After Vitamin D3, Omega-3s, and magnesium, the next best supplement to add to your daily routine would be probiotics (with prebiotics). If you can get your gut healthy, you can make your immune system stronger, which will, in turn, reduce your inflammation. And lastly, add a greens supplement to cover any holes you may have in your diet—which leads to the next thing on the list....

3. Take a good look at your diet.

As you review your diet, pay special attention to your carb, protein, and fat intake.

Carbs: Without getting obsessive about it, you will likely benefit from removing gluten from your diet. Not only will removing it reduce the gut inflammation that comes from processing gluten (and the pesticides sprayed on the crops), but it often leads to cutting out a bunch of junky carbs. Cutting out junky carbs is helpful for everyone, especially if you have Type 2 diabetes.

Protein: Get pickier about your protein targets. Try to hit 0.7-0.8 grams per pound of body weight each day. A palm-size serving of animal protein is the equivalent to approximately 20-25g of protein. Check out my YouTube channel for more suggestions.

Fat: Shift your mindset from cutting out all fats to incorporating healthy ones. Make sure your fat sources come from things like olive oil, avocados and avocado oil, grass-fed butter, and coconut oil. Eliminate hydrogenated oils and seed oils.

Remember, healthy fats are important—they literally make up your cell membranes and assist with the absorption of key vitamins.

4. Experiment with intermittent fasting.

Try to reach a 12-16-hour fasting period three times a week. Of course, the necessary caveats apply here: If you are pregnant or nursing, a teenager, or someone with an eating disorder, then fasting isn't for you. This is also true if you are a female who has difficulty regulating your hormones. (If that describes you, I highly recommend reading *Fast Like a Girl* by Mindy Pelz). Most people I see in my practice are in their fifties or older, so intermittent fasting makes sense for them and helps many of them reach their health goals.

5. Reduce your stress levels.

Add breathwork or meditation to your routine, especially if you have tried the other things on this list and are still struggling with your health and/or sleep. Stress has a huge effect on the body, so a ten-minute practice in the morning or at night can be highly beneficial. Check out my YouTube channel, Dr. Jason Plotsky, for some free resources.

6. Level up your sleep hygiene.

Continuing with what you started in Level One, add in not eating two hours before bed. Then, set a goal to build that up to three hours before bed. From there, challenge yourself not to drink caffeine after 12 p.m. and to avoid alcohol late at night. As you do this, don't skip the basics: Be in bed by 11 p.m. and avoid electronics one hour before bedtime.

7. **Test your mobility and began a weekly practice.**

Use the YouTube link and test your mobility. Score yourself according to the video and start to incorporate a mobility practice into your weekly routine. Use this link for some mobility ideas.

Mobility Test   Mobility Ideas

If you've found five or six items under Level Two that could use some focused effort, then start with Level One, and make sure you're doing those things consistently before you move on to Level Two. The Level One steps will set up a good foundation for higher-level work. Only when you're doing Level One habits consistently should you look at challenging yourself more with Level Two. Once you've nailed the basics in Level One, you will have momentum and have proven to yourself that you can do this! What next?

If you're feeling comfortable with everything in Level Two, then congratulations! You're at an exciting threshold in health. You've got the basics and some of the advanced work done.

The Two-Week Food Challenge

I mentioned changing habits earlier, but I want to provide some detail for those who need a jumpstart on it. The Two-

Week Food Challenge is a hard reset yes, but it yields quick results that may encourage you to keep going. Do the best you can, and keep in mind that this challenge is you ripping off the bandage; you're trying to get rid of everything processed, especially if you feel you're addicted to bread, sugar, or carbohydrates of any stripe. The only way we're going to get an idea of what normal would look like for your body is to do a two-week, no-sugar, no-grains diet. You won't be counting calories; instead, you will:

- Eliminate all alcoholic beverages.
- Cut out all added sugars, including natural sugars.
- Avoid fruits (except berries).
- Eliminate juices, especially those with added sugar, honey, or maple syrup.
- Cut out desserts, cakes, cookies, ice cream, muffins, etc.
- Avoid starchy vegetables like potatoes.
- Cut out bread, pasta, crackers, chips, and similar items.
- Avoid condiments (a sneaky sugar source).

This sounds pretty hardcore, right? It is. But the Two-Week Food Challenge yields the fastest results in the shortest amount of time. This is where knowing if you are a Level One or a Level Two will help make this more approachable, so let's break the challenge down by level.

Preparation (Both Levels)

- Clean out your fridge and pantry.
- Remove all addictive foods from your environment.

(You know your own triggers, whether it's chocolate or chips or muffins.)

Level One

For this level, don't worry as much about getting it perfect; just get rid of the worst stuff first.

- Cut out sodas.
- Eliminate sweets like ice cream or candies.
- Remove anything processed (including all fast foods).
- Don't focus yet on reducing overall food intake/calories, just the types of food.
- Eat some protein at every meal.

Level Two

If Level One feels pretty easy to you, or you want to amp things up, try Level Two and focus on other aspects of your diet as well.

- Eliminate remaining grains.
- Avoid all fruits (except berries).
- Focus on eating non-starchy vegetables.
- Include high protein dairy such as plain Greek yogurt and cottage cheese.
- Eat unprocessed cheeses such as feta, pecorino, or parmigiano reggiano.
- Consume lean protein, including shellfish and eggs.
- Find healthy snack options if you find yourself hungry between meals.

General Tips for Both Levels

This challenge is not easy. Usually, the first three days will end up being the worst, and that's where most people give up. I'm not going to lie—those first three days will suck. If you've been eating a lot of sugar, you're going to experience the ups and downs of going through sugar withdrawal. Salt can come in handy here; when you eliminate sugar and those quick carbohydrates from your diet, your insulin levels will drop, and you'll be letting go of more water. Your need for salt and electrolytes will go up. You can address this with our trusty solution of the daily liter of water and the quarter teaspoon of sea salt, or eat three big dill pickles and five olives each day.

In both the Level One and Level Two versions of the challenge, your focus will be on proteins and fats. You're not trying to reduce your calories; you're just trying to reduce the sugars you're eating and get your carbohydrates in from vegetable sources. We can stabilize the blood sugar with proteins and fats, and that will keep you from having big blood sugar swings.

Sometimes people will treat this challenge like a cleanse, and drastically reduce the amount of food they eat. That's not necessary here. Those first few days will be rough enough, so why add to your misery? If you're addicted to sugar, then probably all you're going to be thinking about is sugar.

Any time we do something hard, we need leverage. We get leverage by thinking about our big goals, or by thinking about the benefits we want to reap. You have to stay focused on your *why* because these first few days in particular will be rough. And you'll have other days, stressful days, where the easier road will be to indulge or give up. That's when your *why* should take center stage in your mind.

Your blood sugar can reset itself in a couple of weeks. Your cravings for sweets will go away in a couple of weeks; it's worth it. If you can sustain it. It's also helpful to plan your meals a few days out; we have seven-day meal plans for people available for this reason.

You can access some sample meal plans here:

The Next Steps

So where does the road go from here? Is there a Level Three?

We're still working on that. From here, the science is much more cutting-edge, and very much still in development. Because the next steps are often so person-specific at this more advanced stage, I can't make any general recommendations in this book. That is why I have created an executive-level health coaching program that you can apply for on my website.

For now, let's look at mindset and environment one last time so when you close this book, you have the complete support you need to get started.

Progress Over Perfection

Try not to let the idea of the checklists or the Two-Week Food Challenge overwhelm you.

Slow down a moment and remember how amazing the human body is. Your work here is as much in reducing stress as it is in changing your habits. Remember back in the stress chapter when we talked about our analogy of the cup and the faucet? It's unrealistic to think you can shut down all the lifestyle stress going into your cup as you make these changes. You won't magically have the perfect lifestyle starting tomorrow.

Instead, recognize where your biggest stressors come from. What things are dripping the most into your cup? How can you slow those down?

Some people look so far forward that all they can see is how far they still have to go on their health journey. What they forget to do is look backward and appreciate how far they've come to get here. That's important, too—don't obsess over perfection; celebrate the progress!

As long as you're working on one or two things, trying to master a skill and form a habit, then you're moving in the right direction. Once you've mastered that, you can go on to the next one or two things. This approach will make breaking down a massive goal like "good health" into much more manageable things to focus on.

My lifestyle is not perfect, and I work on many of these things daily. Most of the people I work with and coach aren't perfect, yet they're still making progress every year.

Your goal is to make things a habit. That's where the focus needs to be, not on perfection and kicking yourself over every little setback. Focus instead on finding ways to easily implement good choices into your daily life.

Motivation vs. Discipline

There is a significant difference between motivation and discipline, as I've touched on before. You may be motivated to try something from one of the checklists for a week or two, but discipline is continuing to do it long-term to see the results you want.

Discipline is a muscle you build through repetition.

Research suggests that performing a task consistently for 21-30 days can make it a habit. To help, start anchoring new habits to existing routines. Having trouble fitting in your mobility exercises? Then start doing them right after your morning walk. Over time, they will become a part of your routine, and you won't rely on willpower alone to get them done.

Building discipline takes time, and it's okay if some tasks on your checklist take longer to master than others. Unlike motivation, which fluctuates, discipline grows through repeated effort and helps you tackle difficult tasks.

One way I practice discipline is through regular cold plunges. Even on some nights when it's incredibly cold and windy, I go out and climb in the tub. Sometimes, I really don't want to do this. I'll say in my head, *Why am I doing this?*

I don't like being cold. In fact, I hate it. So why do I put myself through it?

It's my version of practicing discipline. The more that I do it, the easier it gets.

Fifteen years ago, I would have told you the hardest things for me not to do would be to eat sugar and use hydrogenated oils. Avoiding grains was also tough. I experimented with these changes over longer periods of time to see what might improve in my physiology. That's the only way you will know if something is truly working. Making an effort to improve your sleep hygiene for a week will not be enough to make it a habit. You have to do these things consistently, over and over, one thing at a time. As you master each one, that opens up the path to harder things.

A Wheel of Health

Imagine each of the pillars as spokes in a wheel. Each spoke of the wheel contributes to the stability of the whole. If a spoke is removed, the wheel becomes lopsided. It wouldn't function as well as a wheel with all its spokes.

That wheel is your cumulative health.

As much as it's important to keep up our strengths, it's also important to figure out where we're weakest and shore that up. Doing more exercise won't change a crappy diet. Even if you have a good diet and exercise, it won't undo the fact that your sleep is crappy. If you're doing those three things, but your body's deficient in certain essential minerals or vitamins, then you will still have suboptimal health.

What I try to do for my clients is figure out where the weak points on their wheels are. If something is already a habit, I don't need to focus there because they've already taken care of it. Attacking those weaknesses and spending time and energy there will have the greatest benefit for them.

Give yourself time to nail down and dedicate energy to improving your health. Make it a habit. At the same time, don't get discouraged. If you've been struggling with certain aspects of your health for twenty years, don't expect to do something for twenty days and magically undo the damage. You may not even see the benefits right away. That is the tough part of keeping a long-term mindset; if you focus on the habits, however, things will change over time.

Environment vs. Willpower

As I discussed before, your environment is a powerful player in the establishment of any new habit.

Remember my Type 2 diabetic patient Gordon? He needed to cut out extra breads and sweets, but his wife kept bringing those things home. This forced Gordon to rely on willpower alone, which was very difficult. When his wife stopped buying those things, it was easier for Gordon to stay on track because his environment aligned with his goals.

Your environment can make or break your success. Instead of relying solely on willpower, you need to set your environment up for success. Here's how:

- Eliminate temptations:
  - Remove unhealthy foods: Clear your home of items that can derail your progress, like chips and sweets. If it's not there, you won't be tempted.
  - Grocery shopping: Be mindful of what you buy. Only purchase foods that align with your health goals.

- Embrace supportive surroundings:
  - Engage supportive people: Surround yourself with individuals who support your goals. Communicate your needs to family and friends.
  - Avoid negative influences: Minimize time with those who sabotage or undermine your efforts.

- Ease your access to healthy choices:
  - Prepare meals at home: Cooking at home allows you to control ingredients and portions, supporting healthier eating habits.
  - Create backup plans for exercise: Have indoor exercise options like a gym membership or online workouts to avoid skipping workouts due to weather.

- Change your mindset and self-talk:
  - Positive language: Use encouraging self-talk. Believe in your ability to succeed and remind yourself what you are capable of.
  - Avoid negative language: Catch yourself when you are being negative and reword your language. Have the mindset that you can do hard things and don't let one slip up derail you from your goals.

- Choose commitment over willpower:
    - Focus on discipline: Remember, discipline is more sustainable than relying on willpower alone.
    - Understand your motivation: Know your *why* for achieving your goals and remind yourself of this reason when you feel like giving up.

As you can see, your environment is more than just your physical surroundings; it's your mindset, your community, your plan, and your *why*. When you've got a hold on these things, you'll no longer have to rely on willpower alone.

Now, Do It Forever

This is where you draw the line for yourself. Take another look at our Level One checklist. On a short-term basis, it seems pretty doable, right? Probably. Like I've said, anyone can do anything in the short term.

What if you tried to do it forever?

The food part is probably going to remain the most challenging. Here is also where your answer to the question of interest versus commitment will come into play.

You have to be able to say, "Over the next X number of weeks, this is the number-one thing I'm committed to doing," and mean it. Write it down. If you're in Level One, maybe shoot for two or three weeks. If you're in Level Two, try for thirty days. You want to set these things up as reflexes, where you don't even have to think about doing them.

You want to make them into habits.

Habit Tracking

Some people do really well with habit trackers because they make it easy to see when you are hitting your targets and when you are not. There are even things you can just print out and stick to your fridge, checking off days when you meet your food goals. Achiever-type personalities tend to really like these: Took my supplements, *check*. Went on a walk, *check*. It affirms for them that they're taking the right steps toward a healthier life.

If you're building a new habit, that kind of positive feedback and affirmation is important. You're showing yourself that you both see in front of you what you need to do and that you have the capacity to do it day in and day out. For additional help, you can also download the habit tracker sheet here:

Start to plan things out. Maybe you do this at the beginning or your day or week. Perhaps you make this part of your Sunday evening ritual, looking at the week ahead and all your events and where you have to plot stuff in. As much work as this sounds like, it's going to make your days much easier. Because when it comes to Tuesday, you don't have to decide what you're doing; you already know because you decided earlier in the week what Tuesday's going to be used for. When you get to that day, all you have to do is execute on the plan.

Our goal is to reduce the number of decisions you have to make. That's why having a plan in front of you is so beneficial. You can see it visually as you begin to check things off. Even better is having an accountability buddy or a coach.

Accountability has also been proven to be one of the best tricks toward accomplishing your goals. Not a great exerciser? The best way to change that is to get a buddy. You'll start going to the gym at the same time, or a yoga class at the same time, or meet for your walk at the same time, because you know your partner will be there waiting for you. On the days you don't want to go, your partner helps you. On the days your partner doesn't want to go, you help them. It doesn't have to be a large group of people at all; it works just fine as two people checking in on each other. So make it a priority to engage a buddy today!

I should also add that these habits don't have to be massive. In fact, I really want you to focus on doing the easy things and building them up. Let's think about the easiest thing we can add to your health. Adding is also much easier than subtracting, which is part of why I so often suggest adding more water or starting off with a focus on hydration. If that's all good, then the next thing might be checking that you're getting enough Vitamin D3 and magnesium. What about omega-3? If all of those are good, then look at getting in 150 minutes of movement per week.

Once you can go through your days and routinely check off those three or four things, they'll start to become habits you won't even have to think about anymore.

What you want to do is constantly advance without becoming overwhelmed.

Here's a plan you can follow:

1. Plan ahead and stay accountable.

   - Recognize your personality type: Are you an all-or-nothing person? If so, anticipate setbacks and plan whom you'll call for support when you slip up.
   - Seek accountability partners to help you stay on track.

2. Focus without obsessing.

   - Avoid getting hyper-focused on details to the point of stress.
   - Understand that perfection is not necessary. Consistency and gradual improvement are key.

3. Identify your starting point.

   - Know your *why* and keep it clear. Why are you embarking on this health journey?
   - Identify the area that will have the greatest benefit on your health and start there.

4. Reduce incremental stress.

   - Think of improving your health as unpacking a

backpack while climbing a mountain—remove one stressor at a time.

- Aim for progress over perfection.

5. Create a supportive environment.

- Surround yourself with like-minded individuals who support your goals.
- Control your environment: Make healthy choices when shopping and choose supportive friends.

6. Join a community.

- Engage with others who are also committed to their health goals and willing to put in the hard work.

If you're looking for free resources, please check out my website and my social platforms.

A Few Reminders Before You Go

What makes you actually achieve a goal? Hard work and discipline, certainly, but also the power of community.

In our online community, we post new content regularly, do Q&As, and keep things interesting so that people feel excited to move forward with their goals. We remind each other that being healthy is a lifelong process, and we encourage each other to refocus when we fall off.

If we want our bodies to function at the highest level possible, then it's not what we do in a day or a week that matters. It's what we do consistently over time. I've helped thousands of people in my practice hit their goals and get rid of pain. They've learned how to make lifestyle changes and do things that are hard, all because we've worked together to make doing the hard stuff a habit.

One of the things I love most about my work is being able to watch people year after year. I have a few patients who have been with me ever since I started my practice. It's been such a privilege to get to see them not just progress toward their goals but still maintain a high level of health late into their lives. Many of them tell me they're healthier in their seventies than they were in their sixties. One of my favorite patients, Betty, was telling me on her eightieth birthday how much better she feels now than she did when she was seventy.

And that is another thing that I think people forget: Whether it's by society or by our doctors, we've been told that whenever our bodies feel bad, it's just a part of the aging process and we have to accept it. Sure, things are going to slow down, but there are ways you can forestall that. I've also seen people's negative health situations completely reverse because of their habits.

Habits are powerful. Good or bad, they will dictate your health.

I promise you if you have enough leverage and a big enough *why*, you can change anything in your life.

Putting It All Together

You've taken in a lot of information over the course of this book, and no doubt if you've gotten this far, you're already thinking about all the things you want to implement. What I want you to understand is you don't have to do everything at once.

Everyone's habits are different. Maybe you're looking at this book and feeling overwhelmed with how much you want to change. Maybe you're already doing 70 percent of this stuff, and you're feeling pretty good. Find a balance between taking on too many things and being super-excited to make a meaningful difference in your life.

I love that you're feeling inspired to take action; don't get me wrong! At the same time, though, I want to make sure you don't take on so much that it becomes unsustainable. There will always be higher levels you can aspire to and climb up to. What I want is for you to find where you're at and what sounds like a reasonable next step to challenge yourself with. Maybe that means a two-week food challenge if you're eating a lot of processed foods. Maybe if you don't exercise at all, it's trying to get some exercise in. If you're already eating mostly healthy foods, maybe we can work on cutting out grains and see how your body feels. If you already exercise, then we can shift more toward resistance training.

There's always more we can do, and that's exciting. Why? Because it's going to get us that supercharged immune system, prolong our lives, and give us more energy to do the things we love. The vast majority of people out there are not experiencing a full life, health-wise. We can choose to see that as sad, or as something full of opportunity. There's an area we can work on that will have the greatest effect on our lives—where is that? How can we shift our environments to support this new change? How can we make it sustainable?

Even if you think you have everything handled in terms of your health, there will always be ways for you to push yourself more. I've been working on my own health for years, and I'm still finding things I want to experiment with and keep pushing. I've spoken briefly about my fascination with the biohacking space as well as cold exposure and breathwork. There really isn't a finish line. Isn't that awesome?

That being said, as much as I love nerding-out about health information, I don't want you to just read this book and then not do anything. I want you to put it into action. Each year, think about where you're at and where you could do a little more. Look back on where you've come from and figure out what you're going to do differently in the next year.

For example, last year I did a dry January, consuming no alcohol. That wasn't super-hard for me, but it was something I had to pay attention to. I don't drink a lot, but I like red wine and my wife and I are fairly social people. I just had to tighten that up during that month. Then I tried a fasting regime, like a multi-day fast, to see how my body liked it.

Stay curious. Keep asking yourself what feels good, and what could feel better. And don't be afraid to try new things! I wouldn't have known I could so easily do a dry January if I hadn't attempted it. I wouldn't know whether or not a multi-day fast worked for my body until I actually did one.

At this point, you probably know your reason has to be bigger than you. It ties into your purpose. If you really love an aspect of your life, so much that you're passionate about it, then I can show you how to live healthier so you can do more of that, longer. Anyone can do something for a week. Doing something for thirty days is not as easy—that's why you need a why. You'll rely a lot on your why.

You don't have to be doing everything at once, let alone doing things perfectly. All we care about is improvement and you knowing what the next step is for your journey. That's it. If you're consistent and disciplined enough to continue month after month, you'll get there.

I hope you'll use this book as a resource across many years of your health journey. Maybe during your first year, you implement a few things we discuss; then during your second year, you reread it and find more areas to start improving next. Over time, you'll develop a new set of habits.

I'd also like to underscore this is all a gradual process. I'm not asking you to stop eating bread immediately, cut out all sugar, and then exercise for an hour a day right off the bat. This is much more about establishing a continuum of health.

When it comes to health changes, addition is easier than subtraction. Add water, add supplements, and add in a few more steps than you usually do. Addition is always going to be easier than subtraction, and those three things will make you feel better.

You can make small changes over time that add up and shift your health on a large-scale basis. Again, get rid of the idea that you have to be perfect for this to work. You don't! We can start small. What you're going to do, though, is become consistent and patient. That won't happen overnight.

Keep in mind that you might be in a totally different place health-wise a year from now. Make a plan to revisit this book then. You'll likely glean different ideas out of it on the second reading. It may even spark you to do your own research on a topic that piques your curiosity.

Ready, Set, Go

Now it's time to kick off your health journey. Whether you struggle up a flight of stairs, or you're already walking or working out multiple times per week, the sky's the limit for your fitness.

Remember to check out my YouTube channel where I've recorded videos that dive even deeper into these details, including a video on supplements I recommend. I also have extensive mobility exercises and routines you can watch and follow along with. I've even got a meditation exercise recorded to help you lower stress.

My blog is also a great, free place to read health tips that I post every month. You can find that at www.DrJasonPlotsky.com/blog

At the end of the day, though, action trumps everything else.

You can figure out what you need to do, say all the right things, and know your big, motivating why. What matters most is that you take action and then keep that momentum going.

The magic of the human body, what makes us so incredible, is that this strategy works. Those small changes add up. If you start today with tiny, sustainable changes, where will you be a year from now? What dreams and goals will be within your grasp?

I can't wait to see you achieve them.

References

Asprey, Dave. *The Bulletproof Diet.*

Attia, Peter. *Outlive.*

Chestnut, James. *Eat Well, Move Well, Think Well.*

Clear, James. *Atomic Habits.*

Davis, William. *Wheat Belly.*

DiNicolantonio, James. *The Salt Fix.*

Fogg, B. J. *Tiny Habits.*

Fung, Jason. *The Diabetes Code.*

Fung, Jason. *The Obesity Code.*

Greenfield, Ben. *Boundless.*

Hardy, Benjamin. *Willpower Doesn't Work.*

Hof, Wim. *The Wim Hof Method.*

Longo, Valter. *The Longevity Diet.*

McKeown, Patrick. *The Oxygen Advantage.*

Nester, James. *Breathe.*

Porges, Stephen. *The Polyvagal Theory.*

Ratey, John. *Spark.*

Sinclair, David. *Lifespan.*

Sisson, Mark. *The Primal Blueprint.*

Starret, Kelly. *Built to Move.*

Walker, Matthew. *Why We Sleep.*

About the Author

D r. Jason Plotsky has been in private chiropractic with his wife Cindy since 2003. During this time, he has helped thousands of people get out of pain and implement long-lasting healthy habits. Dr. Plotsky graduated summa cum laude from Palmer College of Chiropractic where he learned about the impact of lifestyle on the prevention of disease and the pursuit of optimal health.

He has travelled all over North America, learning from world experts like Wim Hof, Tony Robbins, and Dr. Joe Dispenza. He also holds certification as a nutrition coach and has completed certifications as a health coach and a high-performance coach.

Dr. Plotsky is still in full-time active practice and resides with his wife Cindy and three boys in Halifax, Nova Scotia. You can sign up for his free newsletter at DrJasonPlotsky.com, and you will find many health tips on his Instagram, Facebook, and YouTube channels.

Hire Dr. Jason Plotsky
to Speak at Your Next Event

If you want your employees and your organization to benefit from greater health, hire Dr. Jason Plotsky to speak at your next corporate meeting, wellness retreat, or training. He will motivate you and your employees to optimize all the ways you can improve your health and enhance your productivity.

Studies have shown that employees take an average of four days off per year in sick time, but they admit to being unproductive an average of 57.5 days a year. That's equivalent to three months a year!

Healthy employees are more productive, and health is often determined by our daily habits. In an overwhelming and complicated industry, Dr. Jason is able to provide clarity and simple direction. Not only do people walk away from the experience they receive in his programs and speeches with a totally different perspective on their health, but they also learn exactly what habits they can implement immediately to create profound changes in their health.

Keynotes

The following keynote presentations are available in an on-line or in-person format, or contact Dr. Jason to tailor a speech that is perfect for your unique needs.

- **Blueprint for Health:** Explore how our lifestyle choices affect preventable diseases and learn how lifestyle stressors affect the body, why we get sick, and how to manage these stressors so we can add life and vitality to our years.
- **Mindset for Longevity:** Learn the importance of creating a vision for your long-term health and how that vision is key to sustainable change. Practice the effective way to set goals for your health through this session and its accompanying worksheets.

Benefits From Your Commitment

- Healthier employees are happier, more engaged, have better energy, are more productive, and operate at full potential.
- Lower health costs mean more money to reinvest in your workforce.
- You'll enjoy a greater connection with your employees. Employees want their employer to care about them and their health and wellness. Focusing on their health and wellbeing proves you are committed to them.

To find out more about our keynote programs, email:

Jason@DrJasonPlotsky.com

Health Coaching
with Dr. Jason Plotsky

Finally make those lifelong, positive changes to your health that will allow you to fulfill all your goals. Work with Dr. Jason one-on-one and he'll help you, step-by-step, go from where you are to where you want to be.

The key to improving your health is knowing how and where to start—where to focus your time and energy. As your health coach, Dr. Jason will offer you solutions to your problems and give you specific actionable steps to keep your progress in motion.

What you get for your commitment and financial investment:

- Our complete pre-coaching health goals assessment to personalize your experience.
- Choice between a six-month or twelve-month program.
- Monthly coaching sessions with Dr. Jason.
- Actionable and clear steps to hit your goals and see results.

- Access to email and text support from Dr. Jason and his team.

Ready to apply? Visit:

www.DrJasonPlotsky.com/high-performance-coaching

Health Retreats

D r. Jason Plotsky has been doing health retreats abroad since 2018 in both Mexico and Costa Rica. He was inspired to create an immersion experience after some of his own most transformative learning experiences. There is something unique and special about taking the time out of your busy schedule to focus solely on yourself. The retreat experiences have previously been tailored to different audiences while mainly focusing on Dr. Jason's 6 Pillars of Health as described in this book. Combining healthy eating with yoga, breath work, mobility drills, beach workouts, and meditation, each day of the health retreat is curated to maximize your day while also providing the rest and recovery your body needs.

Dr. Jason also hosts local events throughout the year. These range from half-day to full-day events focusing on one or more of the Six Pillars. These events are typically hosted in the Halifax, Nova Scotia area.

You can check his website for future dates of retreats and other events at:

www.DrJasonPlotsky.com/retreat

www.ingramcontent.com/pod-product-compliance
Lightning Source LLC
Chambersburg PA
CBHW051243020426
42333CB00025B/3031